Brain Stimulation in Psychiatry

ECT, DBS, TMS, and Other Modalities

WITHDRAWN

D1355595

Brain Stimulation in Psychiatry

ECT, DBS, TMS, and Other Modalities

Charles H. Kellner

Professor, Department of Psychiatry, and Chief, Division of Geriatric Psychiatry, Mount Sinai School of Medicine, New York, NY, USA

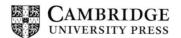

CAMBRIDGE UNIVERSITY PRESS
Cambridge, New York, Melbourne, Madrid, Cape Town,
Singapore, São Paulo, Delhi, Mexico City

Cambridge University Press
The Edinburgh Building, Cambridge CB2 8RU, UK

Published in the United States of America by Cambridge University Press, New York

www.cambridge.org
Information on this title: www.cambridge.org/9780521172554

First published 2012

Printed in the United Kingdom at the University Press, Cambridge

A catalog record for this publication is available from the British Library

Library of Congress Cataloging in Publication data
Kellner, Charles H., 1952–
Brain stimulation in psychiatry : ECT, DBS, TMS, and other modalities / Charles H. Kellner.
   p.   ;   cm.
Includes bibliographical references and index.
ISBN 978-0-521-17255-4 (pbk.)
I. Title. [DNLM: 1. Electroconvulsive Therapy.   2. Deep Brain Stimulation.   3. Mental
Disorders – therapy.   4. Patient Selection.   5. Transcranial Magnetic Stimulation.
6. Vagus Nerve Stimulation.   WM 412]
616.89′122–dc23

                                                                    2012015484

ISBN 978-0-521-17255-4 Paperback

This book is dedicated to my wife, Andrea, with appreciation for her unending patience and support.

Contents

Acknowledgments

I would like to acknowledge the skillful assistance of Rosa Pasculli and Mimi Briggs in the preparation of the manuscript.

Contributors

Ron L. Alterman, MD
Department of Neurosurgery,
Friedman Brain Institute of the
Mount Sinai School of Medicine,
New York, NY, USA

Eran Chemerinski, MD
Assistant Professor,
Department of Psychiatry,
Mount Sinai School of Medicine,
New York, NY, USA

Wayne K. Goodman, MD
Esther and Joseph Klingenstein
Professor and Chair of Psychiatry,
Professor of Neuroscience,
Mount Sinai School of Medicine,
New York, NY, USA

Charles H. Kellner, MD
Professor, Department of Psychiatry,
Chief, Division of Geriatric
Psychiatry,
Mount Sinai School of Medicine,
New York, NY, USA

Chapter 1

Introduction

The field of brain stimulation in psychiatry is advancing at a rapid pace. Practitioners, researchers, and educators have a need to stay informed about the latest advances in these therapeutic modalities. This manual summarizes the information about the brain stimulation techniques currently used for the treatment of psychiatric illness. It covers the scientific basis for the efficacy of each modality, describes the technique itself, and explains the clinical conditions for which each is indicated. Likely future directions for each of the stimulation techniques are discussed.

ECT has by far the longest track record of use as well as the largest medical and scientific evidence base supporting its efficacy and safety. It remains a standard treatment in the psychiatric armamentarium around the world. It is important for psychiatrists to be aware of the most recent advances in technique and clinical indications that allow ECT to be effective and better tolerated than ever before.

DBS is a fascinating brain stimulation modality that has recently crossed into psychiatry from neurology, where its principal use is in Parkinson's disease. While approved currently in psychiatry only for refractory OCD, it is being studied for use in refractory depression, an indication that is likely to greatly expand its use. Because DBS involves direct stimulation of brain tissue, it has promise as a powerful investigative tool in neuroscience.

Transcranial magnetic stimulation (TMS) is a non-invasive brain stimulation modality that has been approved for the treatment of depression in the United States and Canada, as well as several European countries. It is in its clinical infancy and is still only modestly effective for the treatment of depression. It has wide appeal, however, because of its non-invasive nature and excellent safety profile.

Other, less widely used, or experimental, brain stimulation techniques such as vagus nerve stimulation (VNS) and magnetic seizure therapy (MST), among others, are described and assessed as to their likely roles in future clinical practice.

With the citations at the end of each chapter of the manual, the reader will find a concise reference guide to the state-of-the-art of the medical literature for each modality.

Brain Stimulation in Psychiatry: ECT, DBS, TMS, and Other Modalities, Charles H. Kellner. Published by Cambridge University Press. © Charles H. Kellner, 2012.

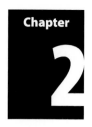

Chapter 2

Electroconvulsive Therapy (ECT): Basic Concepts

Basic Concepts

Electroconvulsive therapy (ECT) is a safe, reliably effective procedure; it requires that the practitioner have a theoretical and practical background to perform it well. Our hope is that this book will assist the practitioner in the application of previously acquired knowledge of ECT. Our intent is that this book should complement the existing, comprehensive texts on ECT, including the report of the American Psychiatric Association (APA) Task Force on Electroconvulsive Therapy (2001) (American Psychiatric Association, 2001), *Electroconvulsive Therapy* by Richard Abrams (Abrams, 2002), and *Electroconvulsive and Neuromodulation Therapies* by Conrad Swartz (Swartz, 2009). *Electroconvulsive therapy: a guide for professionals and their patients* by Max Fink (Fink, 2009) is also recommended.

Our belief is that ECT is a well-standardized procedure that can be learned quite easily. The body of knowledge that the practitioner must master is circumscribed and not overly complex. Of course, as in any clinical endeavor, situations arise that require expert judgment and some modification of standard technique. There is no substitute for clinical experience, and consultation with experts is recommended in difficult cases.

The goal of this text is to provide a practical and useful outline of the basics of the treatment and to assist the reader in developing a well-informed, common-sense attitude to approaching the patient who needs ECT. At all times, technical excellence and patient comfort should be foremost considerations.

Overview

ECT remains the most reliably effective treatment for serious depression (Lisanby, 2007). Its efficacy and speed of response compare favorably to those of antidepressant medications (Husain et al., 2004). For these reasons, it must be considered a mainstream treatment in modern psychiatric practice, not one that is optional or "on the fringe." In the past two decades, there has been a steady

Brain Stimulation in Psychiatry: ECT, DBS, TMS, and Other Modalities, Charles H. Kellner. Published by Cambridge University Press. © Charles H. Kellner, 2012.

increase in ECT research, as evidenced by the growing number of ECT-related citations in the scientific literature. In addition, renewed clinical interest in ECT has led to the growth of professional societies dedicated to the advancement of ECT including the International Society for ECT and Neurostimulation (ISEN, formerly the Association for Convulsive Therapy [ACT]) and the European Forum for ECT (EFFECT), among others worldwide. Innovations in technique (e.g., the electrical dose-titration method of estimating seizure threshold) (Sackeim et al., 1987), the use of ultrabrief pulse stimuli (Sienaert et al., 2009), as well as new information about the use of ECT in catatonia (Fink and Taylor, 2006) and as a continuation/maintenance treatment for affective disorders (Kellner et al., 2006), have been exciting recent developments.

Despite the ongoing barrage of criticism of the treatment (based largely on either outdated or incorrect information), ECT has remained in continuous use since its introduction in Rome in 1938. But modern ECT is so far removed from that primitive procedure that it should hardly be considered the same treatment. Just as it would be unreasonable to equate surgery as performed in 1938 with surgery as performed in 2010, so old-fashioned ECT is now of purely historical interest. The remarkable popularity of the movie *One Flew Over the Cuckoo's Nest* is largely responsible for the continued public perception of ECT as a barbaric, coercive procedure. Two recent books for the lay public, *Shock Therapy: a History of Electroconvulsive Treatment in Mental Illness* by Edward Shorter and David Healy (Shorter and Healy, 2007), and *Shock: the Healing Power of Electroconvulsive Therapy* by Kitty Dukakis and Larry Tye (Dukakis and Tye, 2006) are both informative and factually accurate; they paint a realistic and positive picture of contemporary ECT.

Although ECT is an essential part of psychiatric practice, it remains a very small part. According to data from the National Institute of Mental Health (NIMH), in 1980, approximately 32,000 psychiatric inpatients received ECT in the United States; in 1986, the number increased to approximately 37,000 (Thompson et al., 1994). The current figure of patients who receive ECT annually in the United States is almost certainly greater, although, surprisingly, precise data are unavailable. Hermann et al. estimated that 100,000 patients received ECT in the United States in 1995 (Hermann et al., 1995); Abrams estimated that 1–2 million patients per year receive ECT worldwide (Abrams, 2002).

Health care reform has led to more frequent use of ECT and a greater emphasis on the ability to offer the treatment to outpatients. Because ECT is likely to be more effective than antidepressant medications for many patients (Janicak et al., 1985), it stands to reason that it would be viewed favorably in an increasingly cost- and efficiency-conscious environment.

The old assumption that a course of ECT necessitates being in the hospital is no longer valid. Of course, some patients will be so severely ill as to require hospitalization. Many, however, with adequate family support and close attention to the logistics of treatment, for example, explicit written instructions about concurrent medications, nothing by mouth (NPO) status, proscription of driving, can be safely and comfortably treated as outpatients (Jaffe et al., 1990; Fink et al., 1996).

Because ECT requires specialized knowledge and technical skill, it is likely to be performed by only a small minority of psychiatrists. Thus, local ECT experts, to whom other practitioners refer patients, may be the norm.

Although there may be some controversy about what level of ECT expertise should be required of all psychiatric residents, there can be little disagreement that all psychiatrists should know enough about ECT to make informed referrals to ECT practitioners. Furthermore, the report of the APA Task Force on Electroconvulsive Therapy (American Psychiatric Association, 2001) makes specific recommendations about minimum didactic and practical experiences for psychiatric residents and practitioners who want to be privileged by a hospital to perform ECT.

ECT should be performed only by qualified personnel in an appropriate setting. This setting is generally in a hospital or clinic where access to the equipment and personnel necessary to handle cardiopulmonary emergencies is available. Close cooperation with the staff who provide anesthesia support is essential for optimal ECT. As in all medicine, the goal of scientific and technical advancement remains improved patient care. Our approach to the patient referred for ECT (i.e., the ECT consultation) is quite simple. We require that three questions be answered:

1. Does the patient have an ECT-responsive illness?
2. Does the patient have any medical problems that might require modifications of technique or increase the risks of the procedure?
3. Has appropriate informed consent been obtained?

Each of these questions and many other related issues are covered in subsequent chapters.

Theories of Mechanism of Action

ECT has multiple, profound effects on brain systems, and hypotheses about its mechanism(s) of action are plentiful. Patients and practitioners, understandably, would be comforted by knowing exactly how ECT exerts its therapeutic effects. We are not yet able to explain this in an accurate and comprehensive way. However, rather than settle for a stark "we don't know" response to the question of how it works, it may be more reasonable to invoke one of the better-supported theories of mechanism of action (see below). In truth, we know nearly as much about how ECT works as we do about how antidepressant medications work. A full understanding of how ECT (and other antidepressant treatments) works may need to await a more thorough understanding of the etiology of the major psychiatric illnesses.

Research over the last several decades has provided a wealth of information about specific changes in neurobiology induced by ECT (Sackeim, 1989; Swartz, 2009; Mann, 1998). The classic research of Ottosson (Ottosson, 1960, 1962) using lidocaine-modified ECT helped to establish the seizure as crucial to the efficacy of ECT. The finding that low-dose right unilateral ECT produces suboptimal clinical outcomes despite adequate seizure duration confirmed that not all ECT seizures are equivalent (Sackeim et al., 1987). It appears that both the anatomic location of seizure initiation as well as intensity of the electrical stimulus affect both therapeutic efficacy and cognitive effects (Nobler et al., 2000). A search has begun for more sophisticated measures of seizure therapeutic adequacy other than seizure duration (e.g., postictal electroencephalographic [EEG] suppression) (Nobler et al., 1993; Krystal and Weiner, 1994), but, as yet, no reliable, clinically useful measure has been validated. In short we still lack a definitive understanding of how ECT results in antidepressant and antipsychotic effects. Four main theories are summarized below:

Classical (Monoamine) Neurotransmitter Theory

This theory suggests that ECT works in a way similar to that of antidepressant medications – that it enhances deficient neurotransmission in relevant brain systems. This is a corollary of the classical monoamine depletion theory of depression, a theory that has been updated to include the possibility of a modulatory role for monoamine systems, rather than a simple deficit-adequacy model (Heninger et al., 1996). Specifically, ECT is known to enhance dopaminergic, serotonergic, and adrenergic neurotransmission. Animal studies using ECS (electroconvulsive shock, the term for ECT in animals) have demonstrated increases in dopamine-related behaviors (Fochtmann, 1994). The exact mechanism for this dopaminergic enhancement is as yet unclear; however, it may involve increased dopamine release, receptor changes, and/or changes in the blood-brain barrier (Fall et al., 2000). The fact that ECT has clear antiparkinsonian effects argues strongly for dopaminergic enhancement (Popeo and Kellner, 2009). That ECT also has profoundly antipsychotic effects (and we would expect decreases in dopamine function to be associated with antipsychotic effects) argues against a single theory of increased dopamine availability throughout the brain.

Numerous studies of the serotonin system in both animals (ECS) and humans (ECT) have revealed a complex pattern of changes to pre- and post-synaptic receptors, the serotonin transporter and serotonin metabolites in the cerebrospinal fluid, not all of which are consistent with a simple theory of serotonin enhancement with ECT (Swartz, 2009). For many years, based on animal studies, the serotonin system was believed to be the only monoaminergic system in which ECT had opposite effects from most antidepressant drugs. ECS increases $5\text{-}HT_2$ receptor number, whereas antidepressant drugs decrease $5\text{-}HT_2$ receptor number (Mann and Kapur, 1992). A recent

PET scan investigation found, in contrast to the ECS studies, that ECT reduces brain 5-HT$_2$ receptors in depressed patients (Yatham et al., 2010). These authors speculated, "the ability of ECT to further down-regulate brain 5-HT$_2$ receptors in antidepressant non-responsive individuals may explain its efficacy in those people with antidepressant refractory depression." Rudorfer et al. (1988) demonstrated that 5-hydroxyindoleacetic acid (5HIAA), the major metabolite of serotonin, was increased in the spinal fluid of patients after ECT.

The adrenergic system is also affected by ECT; here, too, numerous preclinical, as well as clinical studies have yielded complex, sometimes contradictory findings. As with other antidepressant drugs, down regulation of beta-adrenergic receptors has been a consistent finding in ECS studies. More recent studies suggest that ECS results in increased cortical norepinephrine transmission as a result of postsynaptic effects (Newman et al., 1998). However, human studies have failed to find consistent alterations in norepinephrine turnover with ECT (Rudorfer et al., 1988).

Other neurotransmitter systems, including glutamate and GABA have been implicated in the mechanism of action of ECT. Studies of glutamate, in both animals and human subjects, have yielded conflicting results. Pfleiderer et al. (2003) showed reduced glutamate with magnetic resonance spectroscopy in the anterior cingulate of depressed patients; glutamate levels normalized with successful ECT. A more recent study showed the opposite in the rat hippocampus, with glutamate levels decreasing after ECS (Dong et al., 2010). Glutamate may be involved in both the antidepressant and the cognitive effects of ECT.

The GABA system has been implicated in the antidepressant and anticonvulsant properties of ECT (Swartz, 2009). Both animal (Ferraro et al., 1990) and human studies (Esel et al., 2008) have demonstrated increases in GABA levels after ECS or ECT. As a major inhibitory neurotransmitter that is measurable in human serum, GABA is likely to be the focus of further investigations of ECT's mechanism of action in the future.

Neuroendocrine Theory

This theory suggests that ECT-induced release of hypothalamic or pituitary hormones results in antidepressant effects. The specific hormone(s) responsible for this therapeutic effect has yet to be isolated. ECT results in release of prolactin, thyroid-stimulating hormone (TSH), adrenocorticotropic hormone (ACTH), and endorphins, among other neurohumoral substances (Kamil and Joffe, 1991). A putative antidepressant neuropeptide, "antidepressin" or "euthymesin," has been theorized to be released from the hypothalamus during the ECT seizure, exerting beneficial effects on mood disorders in a way similar to that in the diabetes/insulin model (Fink and Nemeroff, 1989).

Many investigations have confirmed both the dysregulation of the hypothalamic-pituitary-adrenal (HPA) in melancholic depression and the correction of this abnormality with successful antidepressant treatment, most notably, ECT (Carroll, 1986). The dexamethasone suppression test (DST), the endocrine test that identifies the HPA abnormality, has also been used as a marker of the adequacy of continuation ECT; failure to normalize has been shown to be an indication of the need for ongoing continuation ECT (for review, see Bourgon and Kellner, 2000).

Anticonvulsant Theory

This theory suggests that the antidepressant effect of ECT is related to the fact that ECT itself exerts a profound anticonvulsant effect on the brain. Several lines of evidence indicate that this is so, including the facts that seizure threshold rises (and seizure duration decreases) over a course of ECT and that some patients with epilepsy have fewer seizures after ECT (Griesemer et al., 1997; Sackeim, 1999). ECT has even been used to treat resistant status epilepticus (Lisanby et al., 2001). Neurohormones have been postulated to mediate this anticonvulsant effect. The cerebrospinal fluid of animals receiving ECS is anticonvulsant when given intraventricularly to recipient animals, possibly as a result of endogenous opioids (Holaday et al., 1986). GABA has also been proposed as a key mediator of ECT's anticonvulsant effect (see above).

Neurotrophic Theory

A substantial amount of recent evidence suggests that ECT, like other antidepressant treatments has neurotrophic properties: the effects of ECT, in contradistinction to those of prolonged depression, may be beneficial for the brain. Animal studies show that ECS (the animal analog of ECT) results in increased neurogenesis and mossy fiber sprouting in the dentate gyrus of the hippocampus (Madsen et al., 2000; Lamont et al., 2005; Bolwig and Madsen, 2007). It is possible that neuroimaging techniques, such as magnetic resonance spectroscopy (MRS), may soon be able to provide evidence for neurogenesis in humans after ECT. Preliminary evidence suggests that ECT may lead to increases in neurotrophic factors such as brain-derived neurotrophic factor (BDNF) in depressed patients (Piccinni et al., 2009).

Basics of Electricity

The ECT practitioner should know the following basic facts about electricity in ECT:

Stimulus Characteristics

Modern ECT devices use alternating current that delivers a stimulus in the form of a series of bidirectional square-wave pulses. This is referred to as a brief pulse or ultra brief pulse (when the pulse width is below 0.5 ms) stimulus. Older

ECT devices delivered a sine-wave stimulus. The brief pulse or ultra brief pulse stimulus is more efficient at inducing seizures and consequently can produce seizures with a lower "dose" of electricity. This results in less cognitive impairment. Emerging data are promising that ultra brief pulse stimuli will be much less cognitively impairing, yet preserve efficacy (Sienaert et al., 2010).

Charge

Charge refers to the total number of electrons flowing through a conductor. Many ECT experts agree that the dose of electricity used in ECT should be expressed in terms of charge. The setting dials on some ECT devices vary the charge (by increasing stimulus duration), despite the fact that they are labeled "energy." The equation for charge is

$$\text{charge} = \text{current} \times \text{time}$$

Charge is expressed in millicoulombs (mC).

Energy

Energy adds a term for voltage to the equation for charge. Thus:

$$\text{energy} = \text{voltage} \times \text{current} \times \text{time}$$

Voltage can be thought of as the pressure with which the electrons are "pushed" through the conductor.

By rearranging the above equation with the substitution of an expanded term for voltage

$$(\text{voltage} = \text{current} \times \text{resistance [Ohm's law]}),$$

we arrive at

$$\text{energy} = \text{current}^2 \times \text{resistance} \times \text{time}$$

Thus, as resistance increases, if current and time are kept constant, energy also increases. Because modern ECT devices are mostly of the constant-current type, a patient with a higher resistance will have more energy delivered than a patient with lower resistance treated at the same setting. The constant-current ECT device is designed to increase the voltage automatically (up to a predetermined safe maximum limit) to deliver the desired charge despite high resistance. Because a patient's resistance (impedance) during the delivery of a stimulus is unknown until the stimulus is delivered, settings on an ECT device in terms of joules (J) must necessarily be estimates based on an arbitrary fixed "standard" impedance (e.g., 200 or 220 ohms). Remember that the dial on the ECT device that controls the length of the stimulus is actually setting the charge and only indirectly setting the energy.

Energy is expressed in terms of joules. Note that the number of joules used in ECT is generally considerably smaller than that used in cardiac defibrillation. ECT devices available in the United States deliver an allowable maximum of 101.4 J. Joules may be converted to millicoulombs by multiplying by 5.7 (assuming fixed impedance of 220 ohms and current of 0.8 A).

Impedance may be highly variable between individual patients. The primary contributor to the impedance of the electrical circuit is not the brain, but rather the skin, the underlying scalp soft tissues, and the skull. The contribution of these elements to the interindividual variability of seizure threshold for ECT requires further research (Coffey et al., 1995; Beale et al., 1994; Sackeim et al., 1994; Petrides et al., 2009).

Electrical Safety

The risk of injury to the patient or the practitioner from being shocked is very small. Theoretically, if the patient's impedance is too high, a skin burn at the electrode site can occur. This possibility is virtually eliminated by the provision of electrical self-test features in modern ECT devices, which allow the psychiatrist to check impedance before delivering the stimulus (see section, "Electrode Site Preparation," in Chapter 3). The person delivering the stimulus is at no risk for getting shocked unless he or she actually touches the metal or the conducting surface of one of the stimulus electrodes. The patient's scalp may be touched (e.g., to provide counterpressure on the left side of the forehead during a right unilateral treatment) during the delivery of the stimulus without fear of being shocked. Calls of "Stand clear!" are unnecessary. However, it is prudent to ensure that anesthesia personnel or other personnel do not touch the electrodes during the delivery of the stimulus.

Medical Physiology

Of greatest importance to the clinician are the physiological effects of ECT on the central nervous and cardiovascular systems. As described in later sections, modifications in ECT technique may be required in patients with neurological or cardiovascular disease.

Cerebral Physiology of ECT

Seizure Induction

ECT involves the use of an electrical stimulus to depolarize cerebral neurons and thereby produce a generalized seizure. The more completely generalized the seizure, the more powerful the antidepressant effect is thought to be. The mechanism by which ECT seizures are propagated is not well understood (Enev et al., 2007). However, important differences between bilateral and unilateral electrode placements may result from differing routes of seizure generalization in the brain (Staton et al., 1981).

Ictal EEG

During the initial phase of the induced seizure, EEG activity is variable, consisting of patterns of low-voltage fast activity and polyspike rhythms. These patterns correlate with tonic or irregular clonic motor movements. With seizure progression, EEG activity evolves into a pattern of hypersynchronous polyspikes and waves that characterize the clonic motor phase. These regular patterns begin to slow and eventually disintegrate as the seizure ends, sometimes terminating abruptly in a "flat" EEG (Weiner et al., 1991) (see Figures 4.8a–c in Chapter 4).

Interictal EEG

Transient, cumulative changes also occur in the interictal EEG in response to a course of ECT. Increased predominance of delta activity on interictal EEG is seen as a function of the number of ECT treatments given in a course of ECT and their rate of administration (Fink, 1979). The interictal EEG typically returns to baseline by approximately 1 month following the ECT course in most patients. Generalized EEG slowing has been associated with a positive outcome after ECT (Sackeim et al., 1996).

Other Neurophysiologic Effects of ECT

The ECT seizure is also associated with a variety of transient and benign changes in cerebral physiology, including increases in cerebral blood flow, cerebral blood volume (resulting in a transient rise in intracranial pressure), and cerebral metabolism. The brief rise in intracranial pressure is rarely of clinical consequence, but it is the reason for the historical proscription of ECT in patients with space-occupying mass lesions. Postictally, cerebral blood flow and metabolism are decreased, often for several days after the seizure, and then return to normal levels. Transient disruptions in blood-brain barrier permeability also occur and may account for the short-lived increase in T1 relaxation times observed on brain magnetic resonance imaging (MRI) after ECT (Bolwig et al., 1977; Scott et al., 1990). Well-controlled imaging studies and postmortem examinations in humans, as well as experimental investigations in animals, provide no evidence that modern ECT produces any pathological change in brain structure (Coffey et al., 1991, Devanand, 1995, Devanand et al., 1994).

Cardiovascular Physiology

Cardiac Rate and Rhythm

ECT results in a marked activation of the autonomic nervous system, and the relative balance of parasympathetic and sympathetic nervous system activity determines the observed cardiovascular effects. Vagal (parasympathetic) tone is increased during and immediately after administration of the electrical stimulus; it may be manifested by bradycardia or even a brief period of asystole. This is generally benign and often resolves spontaneously without intervention (Burd and Kettl, 1998). With development of the seizure, activation of the sympathetic nervous system occurs, resulting in a marked increase in heart rate, blood pressure, and cardiac workload. Peripheral stigmata of sympathetic activation may also be observed; they include piloerection and gooseflesh. The tachycardia and hypertension continue through the ictus and generally end along with the seizure. Shortly after the seizure, there may be a second period of increased vagal tone, which may be manifested by bradycardia and various dysrhythmias, including the appearance of ectopic beats. As the patient awakens from anesthesia, there may be an additional period of increased heart rate and blood pressure as a result of arousal and further sympathetic outflow (Welch and Drop, 1989).

Cardiac Workload

The cardiovascular responses during ECT combine to produce an increase in myocardial oxygen demand and a decrease in coronary artery diastolic filling time. Transient electrocardiographic (ECG) changes in the ST segment and T waves are seen in some patients during and shortly following the procedure, although it is unclear whether these findings are related to myocardial ischemia. A direct effect of brain stimulation on cardiac repolarization has been proposed as an alternative mechanism (Welch and Drop, 1989). No corresponding rise in cardiac enzymes has been found to accompany these ECG changes (Braasch and Demaso, 1980; Dec et al., 1985). An echocardiographic study done during and after ECT treatments found transient regional wall motion abnormalities more often in patients with ST segment/ T wave changes in ECG, suggesting a period of demand myocardial ischemia (Messina et al., 1992). The clinical significance of these findings remains unknown.

References

Abrams, R. 2002. *Electroconvulsive Therapy*. New York: Oxford University Press.

American Psychiatric Association. 2001. *Task Force on Electroconvulsive Therapy. The Practice of Electroconvulsive Therapy: Recommendations for Treatment, Training, and Privileging*. Washington, DC: American Psychiatric Association.

Beale, M. D., Kellner, C. H., Pritchett, J. T., et al. 1994. Stimulus dose-titration in ECT: a 2-year clinical experience. *Convuls Ther*, **10**, 171–6.

Bolwig, T. G., Hertz, M. M., & Holm-Jensen, J. 1977. Blood-brain barrier during electro-shock seizures in the rat. *Eur J Clin Invest*, **7**, 95–100.

Bolwig, T. G., & Madsen, T. M. 2007. Electroconvulsive therapy in melancholia: the role of hippocampal neurogenesis. *Acta Psychiatr Scand Suppl*, 130–5.

Bourgon, L. N., & Kellner, C. H. 2000. Relapse of depression after ECT: a review. *J ECT*, 16, 19–31.

Braasch, E. R., & Demaso, D. R. 1980. Effect of electroconvulsive therapy on serum isoenzymes. *Am J Psychiatry*, 137, 625–6.

Burd, J., & Kettl, P. 1998. Incidence of asystole in electroconvulsive therapy in elderly patients. *Am J Geriatr Psychiatry*, 6, 203–11.

Carroll, B. J. 1986. Informed use of the dexamethasone suppression test. *J Clin Psychiatry*, 47, 10–2.

Coffey, C. E., Lucke, J., Weiner, R. D., Krystal, A. D., & Aque, M. 1995. Seizure threshold in electroconvulsive therapy: I. Initial seizure threshold. *Biol Psychiatry*, 37, 713–20.

Coffey, C. E., Weiner, R. D., Djang, W. T., et al. 1991. Brain anatomic effects of electroconvulsive therapy. A prospective magnetic resonance imaging study. *Arch Gen Psychiatry*, 48, 1013–21.

Dec, G. W., Jr., Stern, T. A., & Welch, C. 1985. The effects of electroconvulsive therapy on serial electrocardiograms and serum cardiac enzyme values. A prospective study of depressed hospitalized inpatients. *JAMA*, 253, 2525–9.

Devanand, D. P. 1995. Does electroconvulsive therapy damage brain cells? *Semin Neurol*, 15, 351–7.

Devanand, D. P., Dwork, A. J., Hutchinson, E. R., Bolwig, T. G., & Sackeim, H. A. 1994. Does ECT alter brain structure? *Am J Psychiatry*, 151, 957–70.

Dong, J., Min, S., Wei, K., et al. 2010. Effects of electroconvulsive therapy and propofol on spatial memory and glutamatergic system in hippocampus of depressed rats. *J ECT*, 26, 126–30.

Dukakis, K., & Tye, L. 2006. *Shock: The Healing Power of Electroconvulsive Therapy*. New York: Avery.

Enev, M., McNally, K. A., Varghese, G., et al. 2007. Imaging onset and propagation of ECT-induced seizures. *Epilepsia*, 48, 238–44.

Esel, E., Kose, K., Hacimusalar, Y., et al. 2008. The effects of electroconvulsive therapy on GABAergic function in major depressive patients. *J ECT*, 24, 224–8.

Fall, P. A., Ekberg, S., Granerus, A. K., & Granerus, G. 2000. ECT in Parkinson's disease-dopamine transporter visualised by [123I]-beta-CIT SPECT. *J Neural Transm*, 107, 997–1008.

Ferraro, T. N., Golden, G. T., & Hare, T. A. 1990. Repeated electroconvulsive shock selectively alters gamma-aminobutyric acid levels in the rat brain: effect of electrode placement. *Convuls Ther*, 6, 199–208.

Fink, M. 1979. *Convulsive Therapy: Theory and Practice*. New York: Raven Press.

Fink, M. 2009. *Electroconvulsive Therapy: A Guide for Professionals and Their Patients*. New York: Oxford University Press.

Fink, M., Abrams, R., Bailine, S., & Jaffe, R. 1996. Ambulatory electroconvulsive therapy: report of a task force of the association for convulsive therapy. Association for Convulsive Therapy. *Convuls Ther*, 12, 42–55.

Fink, M., & Nemeroff, C. B. 1989. A Neuroendocrine View of ECT. *Convuls Ther*, 5, 296–304.

Fink, M., & Taylor, M. A. 2006. *Catatonia: A Clinician's Guide to Diagnosis and Treatment*. Cambridge: Cambridge University Press.

Fochtmann, L. J. 1994. Animal studies of electroconvulsive therapy: Foundations for future research. *Psychopharmacol Bull*, 30, 321–444.

Griesemer, D. A., Kellner, C. H., Beale, M. D., & Smith, G. M. 1997. Electroconvulsive therapy for treatment of intractable seizures. Initial findings in two children. *Neurology*, 49, 1389–92.

Heninger, G. R., Delgado, P. L., & Charney, D. S. 1996. The revised monoamine theory of depression: a modulatory role for monoamines, based on new findings from monoamine depletion experiments in humans. *Pharmacopsychiatry*, 29, 2–11.

Hermann, R. C., Dorwart, R. A., Hoover, C. W., & Brody, J. 1995. Variation in ECT use in the United States. *Am J Psychiatry*, 152, 869–75.

Holaday, J. W., Tortella, F. C., Long, J. B., Belenky, G. L., & Hitzemann, R. J. 1986. Endogenous opioids and their receptors. Evidence for involvement in the postictal effects of electroconvulsive shock. *Ann N Y Acad Sci*, 462, 124–39.

Husain, M. M., Rush, A. J., Fink, M., et al. 2004. Speed of response and remission in major depressive disorder with acute electroconvulsive therapy (ECT): a Consortium for Research in ECT (CORE) report. *J Clin Psychiatry*, 65, 485–91.

Jaffe, R., Dubin, W., Shoyer, B., et al. 1990. Outpatient electroconvulsive therapy: efficacy and safety. *Convuls Ther*, 6, 231–8.

Janicak, P. G., Davis, J. M., Gibbons, R. D., et al. 1985. Efficacy of ECT: a meta-analysis. *Am J Psychiatry*, 142, 297–302.

Kamil, R., & Joffe, R. T. 1991. Neuroendocrine testing in electroconvulsive therapy. *Psychiatr Clin North Am*, 14, 961–70.

Kellner, C. H., Knapp, R. G., Petrides, G., et al. 2006. Continuation electroconvulsive therapy vs pharmacotherapy for relapse prevention in major depression: a multisite study from the Consortium for Research in Electroconvulsive Therapy (CORE). *Arch Gen Psychiatry*, 63, 1337–44.

Krystal, A. D., & Weiner, R. D. 1994. ECT seizure therapeutic adequacy. *Convuls Ther*, 10, 153–64.

Lamont, S. R., Stanwell, B. J., Hill, R., Reid, I. C., & Stewart, C. A. 2005. Ketamine pretreatment dissociates the effects of electroconvulsive stimulation on mossy fibre sprouting and cellular proliferation in the dentate gyrus. *Brain Res*, 1053, 27–32.

Lisanby, S. H. 2007. Electroconvulsive therapy for depression. *N Engl J Med*, 357, 1939–45.

Lisanby, S. H., Bazil, C. W., Resor, S. R., et al. 2001. ECT in the treatment of status epilepticus. *J ECT*, 17, 210–5.

Madsen, T. M., Treschow, A., Bengzon, J., et al. 2000. Increased neurogenesis in a model of electroconvulsive therapy. *Biol Psychiatry*, 47, 1043–9.

Mann, J. J. 1998. Neurobiological correlates of the antidepressant action of electroconvulsive therapy. *J ECT*, 14, 172–80.

Mann, J. J., & Kapur, S. 1992. Clinical studies of adrenergic receptor function in depression: Effect of electroconvulsive therapy. *Clin Neuropharmacol.* 15, 675A–676A.

Messina, A. G., Paranicas, M., Katz, B., et al. 1992. Effect of electroconvulsive therapy on electrocardiogram and echocardiogram. *Anesth Analg*, 75, 511–4.

Newman, M. E., Gur, E., Shapira, B., & Lerer, B. 1998. Neurochemical mechanisms of action of ECS: evidence from in vivo studies. *J ECT*, 14, 153–71.

Nobler, M. S., Sackeim, H. A., Solomou, M., et al. 1993. EEG manifestations during ECT: effects of electrode placement and stimulus intensity. *Biol Psychiatry*, 34, 321–30.

Nobler, M. S., Teneback, C. C., Nahas, Z., et al. 2000. Structural and functional neuro-imaging of electroconvulsive therapy and transcranial magnetic stimulation. *Depress Anxiety*, 12, 144–56.

Ottosson, J. O. 1960. Effect of lidocaine on the seizure discharge in electroconvulsive therapy. *Acta Psychiatr Scand Suppl*, 35, 7–32.

Ottosson, J. O. 1962. Seizure characteristics and therapeutic efficiency in electroconvulsive therapy: an analysis of the antidepressive efficiency of grand mal and lidocaine-modified seizures. *J Nerv Ment Dis*, 135, 239–51.

Petrides, G., Braga, R. J., Fink, M., et al. 2009. Seizure threshold in a large sample: implications for stimulus dosing strategies in bilateral electroconvulsive therapy: a report from CORE. *J ECT*, 25, 232–7.

Pfleiderer, B., Michael, N., Erfurth, A., et al. 2003. Effective electroconvulsive therapy reverses glutamate/glutamine deficit in the left anterior cingulum of unipolar depressed patients. *Psychiatry Res*, 122, 185–92.

Piccinni, A., Del Debbio, A., Medda, P., et al. 2009. Plasma brain-derived neurotrophic factor in treatment-resistant depressed patients receiving electroconvulsive therapy. *Eur Neuropsychopharmacol*, 19, 349–55.

Popeo, D., & Kellner, C. H. 2009. ECT for Parkinson's disease. *Med Hypotheses*, 73, 468–9.

Rudorfer, M. V., Risby, E. D., Hsiao, J. K., Linnoila, M., & Potter, W. Z. 1988. Disparate biochemical actions of electroconvulsive therapy and antidepressant drugs. *Convuls Ther*, 4, 133–40.

Sackeim, H., Decina, P., Prohovnik, I., & Malitz, S. 1987. Seizure threshold in electroconvulsive therapy. Effects of sex, age, electrode placement, and number of treatments. *Arch Gen Psychiatry*, 44, 355–60.

Sackeim, H. A. 1989. The unique contributions of ECT to understanding the pathophysiology and treatment of affective disorders. *Convuls Ther*, 5, 207–8.

Sackeim, H. A. 1999. The anticonvulsant hypothesis of the mechanisms of action of ECT: current status. *J ECT*, 15, 5–26.

Sackeim, H. A., Long, J., Luber, B., et al. 1994. Physical properties and quantification of the ECT stimulus: I. Basic principles. *Convuls Ther*, 10, 93–123.

Sackeim, H. A., Luber, B., Katzman, G. P., et al. 1996. The effects of electroconvulsive therapy on quantitative electroencephalograms. Relationship to clinical outcome. *Arch Gen Psychiatry*, 53, 814–24.

Scott, A. I., Douglas, R. H., Whitfield, A., & Kendell, R. E. 1990. Time course of cerebral magnetic resonance changes after electroconvulsive therapy. *Br J Psychiatry*, 156, 551–3.

Shorter, E., & Healy, D. 2007. *Shock Therapy: A History of Electroconvulsive Treatment in Mental Illness*. New Brunswick, NJ: Rutgers University Press.

Sienaert, P., Vansteelandt, K., Demyttenaere, K., & Peuskens, J. 2009. Randomized comparison of ultra-brief bifrontal and unilateral electroconvulsive therapy for major depression: clinical efficacy. *J Affect Disord*, 116, 106–12.

Sienaert, P., Vansteelandt, K., Demyttenaere, K., & Peuskens, J. 2010. Randomized comparison of ultra-brief bifrontal and unilateral electroconvulsive therapy for major depression: cognitive side-effects. *J Affect Disord*, 122, 60–7.

Staton, R. D., Hass, P. J., & Brumback, R. A. 1981. Electroencephalographic recording during bitemporal and unilateral non-dominant hemisphere (Lancaster Position) electroconvulsive therapy. *J Clin Psychiatry*, **42**, 264–9.

Swartz, C. M. 2009. *Electroconvulsive and Neuromodulation Therapies*. Cambridge: Cambridge University Press.

Thompson, J. W., Weiner, R. D., & Myers, C. P. 1994. Use of ECT in the United States in 1975, 1980, and 1986. *Am J Psychiatry*, **151**, 1657–61.

Weiner, R. D., Coffey, C. E., & Krystal, A. D. 1991. The monitoring and management of electrically induced seizures. *Psychiatr Clin North Am*, **14**, 845–69.

Welch, C. A., & Drop, L. J. 1989. Cardiovascular effects of ECT. *Convuls Ther*, **5**, 35–43.

Yatham, L. N., Liddle, P. F., Lam, R. W., et al. 2010. Effect of electroconvulsive therapy on brain 5-HT(2) receptors in major depression. *Br J Psychiatry*, **196**, 474–9.

Chapter 3

Electroconvulsive Therapy (ECT): Patient Selection and Preparation

Indications

The primary indications for electroconvulsive therapy (ECT) are major depression (both unipolar and bipolar types), mania, and schizophrenia (Table 3.1). Catatonia, once considered rare, is re-emerging as another important indication for ECT (Fink and Taylor, 2006). Although typically considered a secondary treatment after pharmacotherapy has failed, ECT is an appropriate initial treatment in some circumstances (Table 3.2). Such "primary use" of ECT is usually compelled by the urgency of the clinical situation; sometimes it is because the patient prefers ECT to other treatment options. The rapidity with which ECT provides symptomatic relief is often a major advantage in urgent clinical situations (Husain et al., 2004; Kellner et al., 2010).

Major Depressive Episode

The most common indication for ECT is major depressive episode, in both unipolar and bipolar disorders. Most studies have found response rates of 80–90% for major depression treated with ECT, with remission rates often only slightly lower (Kellner et al., 2006). Psychotic features and catatonia are markers of a particularly high ECT response rate in major depression (American Psychiatric Association, 2001). ECT may be unique among medical treatments in that symptom severity predicts better outcome; that is, the more severely ill a patient is at baseline, the more likely he/she is to respond well to ECT (Brown, 2007).

Manic Episode

ECT is highly effective in the treatment of the manic phase of bipolar illness. ECT is more rapidly effective than lithium for mania and may be more effective in mixed or agitated manic states (Small et al., 1988). The efficacy of bilateral as compared with right unilateral ECT for mania remains controversial. Some practitioners advocate daily bilateral ECT early in the treatment course for severe

Brain Stimulation in Psychiatry: ECT, DBS, TMS, and Other Modalities, Charles H. Kellner. Published by Cambridge University Press. © Charles H. Kellner, 2012.

Table 3.1. Indications for ECT

Major depressive episode (unipolar and bipolar)
Mania
Mixed affective state
Catatonia
Schizophrenia with prominent affective symptoms
Schizoaffective disorder

Table 3.2. Indications for ECT as a First-Line Treatment

When there is a need for rapid improvement
• Suicidality
• Malnutrition
• Catatonia
• Severe psychosis with agitation
When other treatments are considered more risky
• In the elderly
• In pregnancy
When the patient prefers ECT

mania (Mukherjee et al., 1994). Delirious mania, while rare, is considered by some practitioners to be a primary indication for ECT (Stromgren, 1997).

Schizophrenia

ECT is used for a subset of schizophrenic patients with affective features, catatonia, or a history of previous response to ECT. ECT generally does not alleviate the negative symptoms of schizophrenia. Combination therapy with antipsychotic medication and ECT may synergistically improve psychosis in schizophrenia (American Psychiatric Association, 2001). First episode psychosis, in which it may not yet be clear whether the illness is affective or in the schizophrenia spectrum, often responds very well to ECT (Kellner, 1995).

Other Indications

Both the mood and the motor manifestations of Parkinson's disease often improve with ECT. The treatment is typically used in the later phases of the disease, when patients have become refractory to or intolerant of antiparkinsonian medication. Because it may be a viable alternative to deep brain stimulation, dopaminergic tissue transplantation or pallidotomy for some patients, further study of ECT in Parkinson's disease is warranted (Kellner et al., 1994). Patients with severe depression and co-morbid Parkinson's disease may be particularly good candidates for ECT.

Catatonia, irrespective of etiology, often responds well to ECT (Fink and Taylor, 2006). ECT response rates for neuroleptic malignant syndrome (NMS) are similar to those for dantrolene-bromocriptine therapy; thus, ECT should be reserved as a secondary therapy for this disorder (Davis et al., 1991; Steingard et al., 1992).

The Pre-ECT Evaluation

The goals of the pre-ECT evaluation are to (1) determine whether ECT is indicated, (2) establish baseline psychiatric and cognitive status to serve as a reference point for assessing patient response and cognitive side effects, (3) identify and treat any medical factors that may be associated with an increased risk of adverse effects from ECT, and (4) initiate the process of informed consent (see "Informed Consent" section at the end of this chapter).

Once the indication for ECT has been clearly identified, markers for clinical response should be established. We recommend the use of standardized measures of clinical response during a course of ECT. These include (1) the Hamilton Rating Scale for Depression (HRSD) (Hamilton, 1960); (2) the Montgomery-Asberg Depression Rating Scale (Montgomery and Asberg, 1979); and (3) a self-rating scale, examples of which are the Beck Depression Inventory (Beck et al., 1961), the Carroll Rating Scale for Depression (Carroll et al., 1981), and the Quick Inventory of Depressive Symptomatology-Self report (QIDS-SR) (Rush et al., 2003), for evaluation of depressive symptoms. A baseline (pre-ECT) assessment of cognitive function is needed to monitor the extent of adverse cognitive effects that may develop during the treatment course. We recommend the Mini-Mental State Exam (Folstein et al., 1975) for this purpose. More formal neuropsychological assessment of cognitive function should be considered for selected cases (e.g., patients with preexisting cognitive impairment or patients who are deemed likely to report subjective memory dysfunction).

Of course, a basic medical and psychiatric workup is an essential part of the pre-ECT evaluation. This should include medical history, physical examination, psychiatric history, mental status examination, and limited laboratory evaluation (in selected cases, an electrocardiogram [ECG], a complete blood count, electrolytes, and liver function tests). Young, healthy patients may not require any laboratory evaluation, in accordance with recently liberalized policies governing ambulatory surgical procedures at many institutions (Tess and Smetana, 2009).

Table 3.3. Pre-ECT Evaluation

– Medical and psychiatric history

– Physical examination

– Mental status examination

– Laboratory evaluation (in selected cases)

    Electrocardiogram

    Complete blood count

    Basic or comprehensive metabolic panel

    Other tests specific to patient's medical condition (e.g., digoxin level, theophylline level)

– Anesthesia consultation

– Consider (in selected cases)

    Computed tomography or magnetic resonance imaging of the brain

    Chest X-ray

    Electroencephalogram

A computed tomography (CT) or magnetic resonance imaging (MRI) scan of the brain is sometimes necessary to confirm or rule out a space-occupying lesion or increased intracranial pressure (Table 3.3). If no brain image is obtained, particular attention should be paid to the fundoscopic examination to rule out papilledema. An electroencephalogram (EEG) may be helpful in detecting previously undiagnosed organic brain disease (e.g., toxic/metabolic encephalopathy) and serves as a record of the patient's brain electrical activity before ECT.

Anesthesia consultation is an important part of the pre-ECT evaluation, and cooperation between the ECT and anesthesia teams is essential. Other consultations may be helpful (e.g., neurology, cardiology) if history, physical examination, or laboratory findings suggest that further evaluation is needed. Optimizing the patient's medical status, with the help of these consultants, is an important part of preparing the patient for ECT.

Although there are no absolute medical contraindications to ECT, there are situations of increased risk (Table 3.4). Careful consideration of risks and benefits is critical when the clinician encounters a patient with serious medical illness who is referred for ECT. The report of the American Psychiatric Association (APA) Task Force on ECT (2001) lists situations of substantial risk, including

Table 3.4. Situations of Increased Risk

- Space occupying cerebral lesion
- Increased intracranial pressure
- Recent myocardial infarction
- Recent cerebrovascular accident
- Aneurysm
- Retinal detachment
- Pheochromocytoma

Table 3.5. Common Medical Conditions That May Necessitate Modifications in ECT Technique

- Chronic obstructive pulmonary disease
- Asthma
- Hypertension
- Coronary artery disease
- History of myocardial infarction
- Cardiac arrhythmia
- History of cerebrovascular accident
- Osteoporosis

(1) space-occupying cerebral lesion or other conditions with increased intra-cranial pressure, (2) recent myocardial infarction with unstable cardiac function, (3) recent intracerebral hemorrhage, (4) bleeding or unstable vascular aneurysm or malformation, (5) retinal detachment, (6) pheochromocytoma, and (7) American Society of Anesthesiologists physical status classification of 4 or 5. Some common medical conditions that may contribute additional risk and may require modifications in ECT technique are listed in Table 3.5.

ECT in Specific Medical Conditions

In this section, we discuss the use of ECT in patients with specific medical illnesses. For a review of ECT in the high-risk patient, see Abrams (1989) and Alexopoulos et al. (1989).

Central Nervous System (CNS) Disease

For a complete review of this topic, please see Kellner and Bernstein in Coffey (1993).

Parkinson's Disease

Nearly half of all patients with Parkinson's disease will experience major depression (Brown and Wilson, 1972). A growing literature supports the use of ECT for the treatment of both depression and the Parkinson's disease itself in patients with Parkinson's disease (Andersen et al., 1987). It has been postulated that the dopamine-enhancing effects of ECT are related to its efficacy in the treatment of the motor systems of Parkinson's disease (Fochtmann, 1988). In patients who are taking Sinemet (carbidopa-levodopa) at the time of their ECT, adjustments in dose (typically, decreasing by 50%) may be required to decrease the likelihood of dyskinesias and delirium (Figiel et al., 1991; Rasmussen and Abrams, 1991). Better definition of the role of ECT in the treatment of Parkinson's disease must await further research (Kellner et al., 1994; Popeo and Kellner, 2009).

Dementia

Differentiating dementia from pseudo-dementia in elderly persons is often a difficult task. When dementia coexists with depression, cognitive function may improve after treatment of the depression. However, patients with preexisting dementia who are given ECT may experience transient cognitive worsening (Hausner et al., 2011). These effects can be minimized by modifications in ECT technique, including (1) decreasing the treatment frequency from three times weekly to once or twice weekly, (2) using unilateral electrode placement, (3) using ultrabrief stimulus parameters, (4) titrating stimulus dose to avoid excessive stimulus doses, and (5) minimizing exposure to anticholinergic pre-medications. Also, elderly patients may be particularly sensitive to ECT-drug interactions. ECT to treat the agitation that is often part of the clinical picture of advanced dementia, while likely helpful, remains controversial (Burgut et al., 2010)

Brain Tumor

A transient rise in intracranial pressure is associated with ECT-induced seizures, an effect most likely related to the increase of cerebral blood flow. This increase in intracranial pressure may put patients with space-occupying brain lesions at risk for brain herniation. The presence of a brain tumor, once an absolute contraindication to ECT, is now no longer thought of as such. Although clearly one of the most significant risks, not all brain tumors are equally problematic (Maltbie et al., 1980). Large edematous tumors causing mass effect are clearly extremely dangerous. However, small calcified meningiomas without associated edema probably pose little risk (Abrams, 2002; Goldstein and Richardson, 1988; Kellner et al., 1991a; McKinney et al., 1998). Neurosurgical consultation should be considered in patients with brain tumors referred for ECT.

Stroke

Stroke related to ECT is a very rare event (Lee, 2006). Patients who have had a recent hemorrhagic stroke may be at risk for rebleeding during ECT. There is little information about the risks of ECT to patients who have had recent ischemic strokes. Generally, withholding ECT for a period of weeks to months is recommended if the patient has had a stroke. However, this delay must be weighed against the severity of the psychiatric illness itself. Extremes of blood pressure, both hyper- and hypotension, should be avoided during ECT in stroke patients. The use of intravenous antihypertensives during ECT may be helpful in safely managing some cases.

Epilepsy

Patients with concurrent epilepsy and depression can be safely treated with ECT. It is recommended that epileptic patients continue to receive their anticonvulsant medications during the course of ECT (Abrams, 2002). The rise in seizure threshold that accompanies ECT may actually reduce the frequency of spontaneous seizures in patients with epilepsy (Dubovsky, 1986; Sackeim et al., 1983; Schnur et al., 1989; Griesemer et al., 1997). ECT has been used as a treatment for status epilepticus (Kamel et al., 2010; Cline and Roos, 2007). Consideration may be given to adjusting anticonvulsant medication during a course of ECT if eliciting adequate seizures becomes difficult.

Cardiovascular Disease

Myocardial Infarction/Ischemic Heart Disease

Although rare, cardiac complications during ECT represent the most common cause of fatality associated with the treatment (Zielinski et al., 1993). The catecholamine surge and subsequent hypertension and tachycardia that accompany ECT-induced seizures may put patients with prior cardiac disease at risk for myocardial ischemia. Also, patients who have had a recent myocardial infarction may be at risk for further myocardial damage. The use of intravenous beta blockers, nitrates and other antihypertensive agents and careful attention to oxygenation are important risk-reducing strategies in this population. We recommend the use of labetalol (5–20 mg IV) or esmolol (5–60 mg IV) for patients with a history of hypertension and/or tachycardia if there is concern about their ability to tolerate the hemodynamic effects of ECT safely. An alternative strategy is to treat patients with coronary artery disease with nitroglycerin, either before the procedure (transdermally or sublingually) or during the procedure (intravenously). Also, regularly prescribed cardiac medications (e.g., antihypertensives or digoxin) should be taken with a small sip of water 2 hours before ECT. (See also section, "Cardiovascular Medications," in this chapter.)

Arrhythmias

To protect against bradyarrhythmia, anticholinergic medication (e.g., glycopyrrolate 0.2 mg IV or atropine 0.4 mg IV) may be given before each ECT. Anticholinergic premedication is recommended whenever stimulus dose titration is performed, particularly in patients receiving beta-blockers. Significant tachyarrhythmias may be treated with intravenous beta-blockers, as previously discussed. Transient benign hypertension, tachycardia, and premature ventricular contractions may occur for several minutes following ECT. These arrhythmias tend to resolve spontaneously and to have little clinical significance. Therefore, unless these conditions are sustained or deemed particularly severe, close observation may be the only necessary action.

Other Medical Conditions

Pulmonary Disease

Patients with preexisting chronic obstructive pulmonary disease or asthma should receive their inhalant bronchodilators before each ECT treatment. Theophylline should be avoided or kept in the low therapeutic range to prevent prolonged seizures or status epilepticus (Schak et al., 2008).

HIV and AIDS

Severe depression associated with human immunodeficiency virus (HIV) and acquired immunodeficiency syndrome (AIDS) has been reported to respond to ECT (Schaerf et al., 1989). It is particularly important to rule out increased intracranial pressure at the time of ECT, because these patients are prone to developing intracranial masses. Kessing et al. (1994) reported successful treatment of HIV-induced stupor with ECT. AIDS-related mania and psychosis may also be indications for ECT.

Pregnancy

ECT has been used safely during all trimesters of pregnancy. ECT may be preferred over psychopharmacological methods because of the brief exposure of the fetus to pharmacological agents during ECT, in comparison to the prolonged exposure to potentially teratogenic agents during the course of a pregnancy. Fetal monitoring is recommended in cases of high-risk pregnancy, and the rapid availability of an obstetric consultant is prudent (Abrams, 2002; Anderson and Reti, 2009).

Neuroleptic Malignant Syndrome

The response rate to ECT is equal to that of pharmacological treatment in patients with NMS (Davis et al., 1991). We recommend ECT in cases in which pharmacological treatment has failed. Other authors believe that aggressive treatment with ECT, similar to that recommended for catatonic patients, is appropriate for patients with NMS (Trollor and Sachdev, 1999; Fink, 1994). Patients with NMS should not receive neuroleptics during ECT.

Gastrointestinal Disorders

Pretreatment with histamine-2 (H_2) blockers, metoclopramide, or sodium citrate is usually sufficient aspiration prophylaxis for most patients with clinically significant gastroesophageal reflux. This strategy may reduce the need for intubation in many cases. Anesthesiologists may elect to intubate patients who have severe reflux disease or those who have a known history of incompetent gastroesophageal sphincters (Tess and Smetana, 2009).

Musculoskeletal Disorders

Appropriate muscle relaxation virtually eliminates risk of fracture during ECT, even in patients with fragile bones (e.g., osteoporosis or recent fracture). However, in patients with severe osteoporosis, it may be advisable to use the higher dose range of 1.0–1.50 mg/kg of succinylcholine to ensure complete muscular blockade. It is also advisable not to use the cuffed-limb method in these cases. Patients with any loose or fractured teeth or with a history of temporomandibular joint disease should have these conditions stabilized before ECT.

Concurrent Medications

A careful evaluation of the patient's concurrent medications is required before ECT. In this section, we review the interactions of psychotropic and other medications with ECT. (See Haskett and Loo, 2010; and Kellner et al., 1991b for more in-depth reviews.) Discontinuation before ECT is required for some agents, whereas modified dosing is recommended for other agents.

Psychotropic Medications

In the past it was recommended that most psychotropic medications be tapered and discontinued before beginning ECT. Nowadays, practitioners are much more liberal in combining ECT and psychotropic medications. This is due to accumulating evidence of additive efficacy with some antidepressants, as well as safety data for many drugs combined with ECT (Lauritzen et al., 1996; Sackeim et al., 2009).

Antipsychotic medication, which may act synergistically with ECT in the treatment of psychotic patients, has for a long time been co-prescribed with ECT. We review below the major categories of psychotropic medications and their interactions with ECT.

Lithium

Recent data suggest that the coadministration of lithium and ECT is relatively safe and that earlier warnings about the combination were overly conservative (Dolenc and Rasmussen, 2005). Nonetheless, the combination has been associated with the development of delirium or prolonged seizures (Weiner et al., 1980). The transient increase in permeability of the blood-brain barrier following ECT (Bolwig et al., 1977) has been proposed as a possible mechanism by which increased concentrations of lithium can enter the CNS. In general, it is advisable to hold lithium for at least 24 hours before ECT, so that patients can be treated with lithium blood levels at the lower end of the therapeutic range.

Antidepressants

The combination of ECT and antidepressant medications, once frowned upon, is now encouraged, both because newer generation antidepressants are safer and because there is accumulating evidence for antidepressant synergy (Sackeim et al., 2009) and possibly enhanced relapse prevention. While some question the practice of continuing previously "ineffective" antidepressants during ECT, in many cases antidepressants have not been completely ineffective and it may be possible to continue an agent that has provided some symptom relief. There is also the possibility that an agent that was not "powerful" enough to treat an acute depressive episode may still confer some relapse prevention benefit in the period after remission with ECT (van den Broek et al., 2006). If a patient begins an acute course of ECT on no antidepressant medication, some practitioners believe that an agent should be started before the end of the acute course of ECT, so that the patient is not left unprotected (i.e., without therapeutic blood levels) when ECT is stopped. The agent may be either one that has been partially effective in the past, or one that is new for the patient. The newer selective serotonin reuptake inhibitors (SSRIs) and serotonin-norepinephrine reuptake inhibitors (SNRIs) pose less cardiac risk when given with ECT than the older tricyclic antidepressants (TCAs). In practice, the combination of these agents and ECT has become widespread.

While TCAs are much less commonly used than in the past, when they are used, there is still concern about cardiovascular effects of interactions between these antidepressants and ECT or the anesthetic agents used during the procedure. The issue of potential adverse effects of tricyclic antidepressants (TCAs) given in conjunction with ECT has generated a plethora of case reports and small case series (Pritchett et al., 1993). Discontinuance of a TCA shortly before beginning ECT may be particularly problematic (Raskin, 1984).

The use of monoamine oxidase inhibitors (MAOIs) in patients receiving ECT remains somewhat controversial, although here, too, there has been a trend to regard the combination more favorably. A critical reading of the literature suggests that the combination is not as risky as once thought (Dolenc et al., 2004). It has been recommended in the anesthesia literature that MAOIs be discontinued up to 2 weeks before elective surgery or ECT. Case reports describe hyper- and hypotension, fever, hyperreflexia, seizures, and hepatotoxicity in patients receiving general anesthesia while taking MAOIs (Jenkins and Graves, 1965). Investigators have documented the safety of ECT in patients receiving chronic MAOI therapy (el-Ganzouri et al., 1985). Because of these conflicting reports, clinicians will have to weigh the risks and benefits of proceeding with ECT in patients taking MAOIs. The newer transdermal delivery form of the MAOI selegiline has been reported to be safe in conjunction with ECT (Horn et al., 2010).

Benzodiazepines

In addition to raising the seizure threshold, benzodiazepines may also decrease the intensity or generalization of the ECT seizure. They may also shorten seizure duration, and their use may increase the number of ECT treatments required for recovery (Stromgren et al., 1980). Pettinati et al. (1990) carried out a comprehensive study of the combined use of benzodiazepines and ECT. They found a significant relationship between therapeutic failure of unilateral ECT and concomitant benzodiazepine use. This lack of efficacy may have been related to the increase in seizure threshold caused by the concurrent benzodiazepines and the low stimulus dosing techniques used. The authors recommended discontinuing benzodiazepines before unilateral ECT is given. This interaction is likely less important when bilateral or high-dose unilateral ECT is used. We believe it is prudent to taper and/or discontinue benzodiazepines before ECT, if possible. However, it is quite permissible to continue low or moderate dose benzodiazepines, if anxiety is a troublesome symptom for the patient. Certainly, if anxiety about the procedure itself might jeopardize the treatment course, the patient may be given benzodiazepines, even on the morning of treatment. We recommend the use of 0.5 mg or 1 mg lorazepam sublingual, approximately 30 minutes before ECT to treat pre-procedure anxiety. For patients who have been taking long half-life benzodiazepines, such as clonazepam, it may be advisable to switch to a shorter half-life drug, such as lorazepam, before starting ECT. This way, benzodiazepine blood levels will be lower at the time of ECT, after the prior evening's dose.

Anticonvulsants

Similar to benzodiazepines, anticonvulsants also raise the seizure threshold and may theoretically interfere with the efficacy of ECT. In patients with epilepsy, anticonvulsants should be continued during a course of ECT. Consideration may be given to adjusting dosage or type of anticonvulsant if it becomes difficult to elicit adequate seizures. Anticonvulsants prescribed for psychiatric indications should usually be tapered and discontinued before beginning ECT. A recent report suggests that concomitant treatment with an anticonvulsant may require longer ECT treatment courses (Virupaksha et al., 2010). There is, as yet, no consensus about whether or not ECT and anticonvulsants may have additive or synergistic effects (Sienaert and Peuskens, 2007; Rubner et al., 2009).

Neuroleptics

Neuroleptics have long been regarded as synergistic with ECT in the treatment of psychotic symptoms. It has been speculated that this effect may be related to their lowering of the seizure threshold (Coffey et al., 1995), although this is far from certain. Low-potency neuroleptics (e.g., chlorpromazine) have been reported to cause hypotensive reactions when given with ECT (Grinspoon and Greenblatt, 1963). High-potency neuroleptics (e.g., haloperidol or fluphenazine) are considered safe when used concurrently with ECT. This combination is indicated particularly in the treatment of psychotic depression. Also, when ECT is used to treat schizophrenia, the combination of ECT and antipsychotic medications may be more effective than ECT alone (American Psychiatric Association 2001).

Atypical Neuroleptics

Atypical or "second generation" neuroleptics are now routinely combined with ECT and the combination is not thought to involve significantly increased risk. Additive or synergistic benefit is likely, as it is with first generation drugs.

Numerous reports document the safety of clozapine with ECT, although special attention to the control of heart rate may be required (Klapheke, 1993). Risperidone and paliperidone have also been used safely with ECT (Farah et al., 1995; Masdrakis et al., 2011).

Psychotropic Medications during Continuation/Maintenance ECT

ECT Most patients are treated with combined medication-ECT strategies during the maintenance phase; however, controlled data are lacking for the development of useful guidelines in this area (Lisanby et al., 2008). Combined antidepressant and ECT treatment should be considered in patients who have responded to acute-phase ECT but have a history of frequent and severe relapses. These patients may discontinue their lithium, anticonvulsants, and benzodiazepines 12–36 hours before each continuation/maintenance ECT and resume them after their ECT. Tapering/discontinuation regimens should be individualized with the aim of reducing the drug level, while paying attention to the possible development of withdrawal symptoms.

Other Agents

Cardiovascular medications

Patients should receive their routine antihypertensive and antianginal medications with a small sip of water approximately 2 hours before ECT. Transdermal nitrates should be in place at least 30 minutes before treatment. Medications that should be avoided before ECT include diuretics (because of the increased risk of incontinence, or, rarely, bladder rupture in patients with a full bladder), reserpine (because of the risk of hypotension and death), and lidocaine (because of its potent anticonvulsant properties).

Hypoglycemics

For patients with diabetes, adjustments in the dosage of insulin and oral hypoglycemics may be required on the morning of ECT because of the overnight fast. Holding the morning insulin dose until after the patient has had breakfast is the usual approach. In severe diabetic patients with a propensity toward ketoacidosis, half of the patient's usual morning dose of insulin may be given with running intravenous dextrose before ECT; this, however, is rarely required (Rasmussen et al., 2006). Consultation with an endocrinologist may be helpful.

Antiasthmatics

Steroids and β-adrenergic agonists should be given before ECT as required to prevent bronchoconstriction. Because of an association with prolonged seizures during ECT, theophylline should be stopped before ECT in most cases. If theophylline is medically required, blood levels should be monitored closely during a course of ECT and kept in the low therapeutic range (Rasmussen and Zorumski, 1993; Schak et al., 2008).

Glaucoma Medications

Patients should receive their glaucoma eye drops before ECT because of the transient increase in intraocular pressure during the procedure. The prominent caveat is that ECT patients should not receive echothiophate (an irreversible cholinesterase inhibitor) because of the risk of prolonged apnea in patients given succinylcholine.

Gastrointestinal medications

Patients with peptic ulcer disease or gastroesophageal reflux disease (GERD) should receive their H_2 blocker or metoclopramide with a sip of water at least

Table 3.6. Morning Medications That Should Be Given Before ECT

Medication	Exclusions
Antihypertensives	Diuretics
Antianginals, antiarrhythmics, digoxin	Lidocaine
Anti-gastric reflux agents	
Glaucoma eyedrops	Echothiophate
Bronchodilators	Theophylline

2 hours before ECT. Sodium citrate (30 cc po) may be given immediately before treatment to neutralize any acid remaining in the stomach.

Anticoagulant medications

Anticoagulants have been used safely during ECT. Coagulation times should be followed during the course of ECT (Tancer and Evans, 1989; Petrides and Fink, 1996; Mehta et al., 2004).

Most other medications can be held until 1–2 hours following each ECT, unless the medication is clearly physiologically protective for the patient during the treatment (Table 3.6).

Informed Consent

Obtaining informed consent from the patient and his or her family is an essential part of the pre-ECT workup. Informed consent requires (1) the provision of adequate information, (2) a patient who is capable of understanding and acting intelligently upon such information, and (3) the opportunity to provide consent in the absence of coercion (American Psychiatric Association 2001, pp. 97–8). This APA report contains an excellent four-page sample informed-consent document. The ECT practitioner should ensure that the ECT consent conforms to all applicable laws, statutes, and hospital policies. Essential information to be included for ECT informed consent includes the following items:

- The indication for ECT
- The effectiveness of ECT for the condition
- Description of the procedure itself
- Routine side effects
- More rare adverse events (e.g., major anesthetic complication)
- Any condition that may place the patient at increased risk

The patient should understand that consent can be withdrawn at any point and should know whom to contact with questions during the treatment course. The patient should be cautioned that major personal or financial decisions should not be made during or immediately after a course of ECT. The patient probably should not drive until the cognitive effects of ECT have largely resolved and, in the case of continuation/maintenance ECT, until 24 hours after treatment.

Consent for the Depressed Patient

Self-disparagement and uncertainty often make treatment decisions difficult for depressed patients. Educating family members is invaluable in helping the depressed patient decide whether to receive ECT. Educational videotapes, provided through each of the major ECT device manufacturers and available from other sources, are often very helpful.

Involuntary ECT

As with any other medical procedure, informed consent for ECT may need to be waived in acute emergencies. ECT may be a lifesaving procedure for acutely suicidal, catatonic, or dangerously malnourished patients. For these patients, and for any patients who lack capacity to provide consent, some form of substituted consent (with surrogate decision makers) is required, as defined by local jurisdiction.

References

Abrams, R. 1989. ECT in the high-risk patient. *Convuls Ther*, 5, 1–2.

Abrams, R. 2002. *Electroconvulsive Therapy*. New York: Oxford University Press.

Alexopoulus, G. S., Young, R. C., & Abrams, R. C. 1989. ECT in the high-risk geriatric patient. *Convuls Ther*, 5, 75–81.

American Psychiatric Association. 2001. *Task Force on Electroconvulsive Therapy. The Practice of Electroconvulsive Therapy: Recommendations for Treatment, Training, and Privileging*. Washington, DC: American Psychiatric Association.

Andersen, K., Balldin, J. Gottfries, C. G., et al. 1987. A double-blind evaluation of electroconvulsive therapy in Parkinson's disease with "on-off" phenomena. *Acta Neurol Scand*, 76, 191–9.

Anderson, E. L., & Reti, I. M. 2009. ECT in pregnancy: a review of the literature from 1941 to 2007. *Psychosom Med*, 71, 235–42.

Beck, A. T., Ward, C. H., Mendelson, M., Mock, J., & Erbaugh, J. 1961. An inventory for measuring depression. *Arch Gen Psychiatry*, 4, 561–71.

Bolwig, T. G. Hertz, M. M., Paulson, O. B., Spotoft, H., & Rafaelsen, O. J. 1977. The permeability of the blood-brain barrier during electrically induced seizures in man. *Eur J Clin Invest*, 7, 87–93.

Brown, G. L., & Wilson, W. P. 1972. Parkinsonism and depression. *South Med J*, 65, 540–5.

Brown, W. A. 2007. Treatment response in melancholia. *Acta Psychiatr Scand Suppl*, 125–9.

Burgut, F. T., Popeo, D., & Kellner, C. H. 2010. ECT for agitation in dementia: is it appropriate? *Med Hypotheses*, 75, 5–6.

Carroll, B. J., Feinberg, M., Smouse, P. E., Rawson, S. G., & Greden, J. F. 1981. The Carroll rating scale for depression. I. Development, reliability and validation. *Br J Psychiatry*, 138, 194–200.

Cline, J. S., & Roos, K. 2007. Treatment of status epilepticus with electroconvulsive therapy. *J ECT*, 23, 30–2.

Coffey, C. E. 1993. *The Clinical Science of Electroconvulsive Therapy*. Washington, DC: American Psychiatric Press.

Coffey, C. E., Lucke, J., Weiner, R. D., Krystal, A. D., & Aque, M. 1995. Seizure threshold in electroconvulsive therapy: I. Initial seizure threshold. *Biol Psychiatry*, 37, 713–20.

Davis, J. M., Janicak, P. G., Sakkas, P., Gilmore, C., & Wang, Z. 1991. Electroconvulsive therapy in the treatment of the neuroleptic malignant syndrome. *Convuls Ther*, 7, 111–20.

Dolenc, T. J., Habl, S. S., Barnes, R. D., & Rasmussen, K. G. 2004. Electroconvulsive therapy in patients taking monoamine oxidase inhibitors. *J ECT*, 20, 258–61.

Dolenc, T. J., & Rasmussen, K. G. 2005. The safety of electroconvulsive therapy and lithium in combination: a case series and review of the literature. *J ECT*, 21, 165–70.

Dubovsky, S. L. 1986. Using electroconvulsive therapy for patients with neurological disease. *Hosp Community Psychiatry*, 37, 819–25.

el-Ganzouri, A. R., Ivankovich, A. D., Braverman, B., & McCarthy, R. 1985. Monoamine oxidase inhibitors: should they be discontinued preoperatively? *Anesth Analg*, 64, 592–6.

Farah, A., Belae, M. D., & Kellner, C. H. 1995. Risperidone and ECT combination therapy: a case series. *Convuls Ther*, 11, 280–2.

Figiel, G. S., Hassen, M. A., Zorumski, C., et al. 1991. ECT-induced delirium in depressed patients with Parkinson's disease. *J Neuropsychiatry Clin Neurosci*, 3, 405–11.

Fink, M. 1994. Indications for the use of ECT. *Psychopharmacol Bull*, 30, 269–75; discussion 276–80.

Fink, M., & Taylor, M. A. 2006. *Catatonia: A Clinician's Guide to Diagnosis and Treatment*. Cambridge: Cambridge University Press.

Fochtmann, L. 1988. A mechanism for the efficacy of ECT in Parkinson's disease. *Convuls Ther*, 4, 321–7.

Folstein, M. F., Folstein, S. E., & McHugh, P. R. 1975. "Mini-mental state". A practical method for grading the cognitive state of patients for the clinician. *J Psychiatr Res*, 12, 189–98.

Goldstein, M. Z., & Richardson, C. 1988. Meningioma with depression: ECT risk or benefit? *Psychosomatics*, 29, 349–51.

Griesemer, D. A., Kellner, C. H., Beale, M. D., & Smith, G. M. 1997. Electroconvulsive therapy for treatment of intractable seizures. Initial findings in two children. *Neurology*, 49, 1389–92.

Grinspoon, L., & Greenblatt, M. 1963. Pharmacotherapy combined with other treatment methods. *Compr Psychiatry*, **18**, 256–62.

Hamilton, M. 1960. A rating scale for depression. *J Neurol Neurosurg Psychiatry*, **23**, 56–62.

Haskett, R.F., & Loo, C. 2010. Adjunctive psychotropic medications during electroconvulsive therapy in the treatment of depression, mania, and schizophrenia. *J ECT*, **26**, 196–201.

Hausner, L., Damian, M., Sartorius, A., & Frolich, L. 2011. Efficacy and cognitive side effects of electroconvulsive therapy (ECT) in depressed elderly inpatients with coexisting mild cognitive impairment or dementia. *J Clin Psychiatry*, **72**, 91–7.

Horn, P. J., Reti, I., & Jayaram, G. 2010. Transdermal selegiline in patients receiving electroconvulsive therapy. *Psychosomatics*, **51**, 176–8.

Husain, M. M., Rush, A. J., Fink, M., et al. 2004. Speed of response and remission in major depressive disorder with acute electroconvulsive therapy (ECT): a consortium for research in ECT (CORE) report. *J Clin Psychiatry*, **65**, 485–91.

Jenkins, L. C., & Graves, H. B. 1965. Potential hazards of psychoactive drugs in association with anaesthesia. *Can Anaesth Soc J*, **12**, 121–8.

Kamel, H., Cornes, S. B., Hedge, M., Hall, S. E., & Josephson, S. A. 2010. Electroconvulsive therapy for refractory status epilepticus: a case series. *Neurocritical Care*, **12**, 204–10.

Kellner, C. H. 1995. Is ECT the treatment of choice for first-break psychosis? *Convuls Ther*, **11**, 155–7.

Kellner, C. H., Beale, M. D., Pritchett, J. T., Bernstein, H. J., & Burns, C. M. 1994. Electroconvulsive therapy and Parkinson's disease: the case for further study. *Psychopharmacol Bull*, **30**, 495–500.

Kellner, C. H., Burns, C. M., Bernstein, H. J., Monroe, R. R., Jr., & George, M. S. 1991a. Safe administration of ECT in a patient with a calcified frontal mass. *J Neuropsychiatry Clin Neurosci*, **3**, 353–4.

Kellner, C.H., Nixon, D.W., & Bernstein, H.J. 1991b. ECT-drug interactions: a review. *Psychopharmacol Bull*, **27**, 595–609.

Kellner, C. H., Knapp, R., Husain, M. M., et al. 2010. Bifrontal, bitemporal and right unilateral electrode placement in ECT: randomised trial. *Br J Psychiatry*, **196**, 226–34.

Kellner, C. H., Knapp, R. G., Petrides, G., et al. 2006. Continuation electroconvulsive therapy vs pharmacotherapy for relapse prevention in major depression: a multisite study from the Consortium for Research in Electroconvulsive Therapy (CORE). *Arch Gen Psychiatry*, **63**, 1337–44.

Kessing, L., Labianca, J. H., & Bolwig, T. G. 1994. HIV-induced stupor treated with ECT. *Convuls Ther*, **10**, 232–5.

Klapheke, M. M. 1993. Combining ECT and antipsychotic agents: benefits and risks. *Convuls Ther*, **9**, 241–55.

Lauritzen, L., Odgaard, K., Clemmesen, L., et al. 1996. Relapse prevention by means of paroxetine in ECT-treated patients with major depression: a comparison with imipramine and placebo in medium-term continuation therapy. *Acta psychiatrica Scandinavica*, **94**, 241–51.

Lee, K. 2006. Acute embolic stroke after electroconvulsive therapy. *J ECT*, **22**, 67–9.

Lisanby, S. H., Sampson, S., Husain, M. M., et al. 2008. Toward individualized post-electroconvulsive therapy care: piloting the Symptom-Titrated, Algorithm-Based Longitudinal ECT (STABLE) intervention. *J ECT*, 24, 179–82.

Maltbie, A. A., Wingfield, M. S., Volow, M. R., et al. 1980. Electroconvulsive therapy in the presence of brain tumor. Case reports and an evaluation of risk. *J Nerv Ment Dis*, 168, 400–5.

Masdrakis, V. G., Tzanoulinos, G., Markatou, M., & Oulis, P. 2011. Cardiac safety of the electroconvulsive therapy-paliperidone combination: a preliminary study. *Gen Hosp Psychiatry*, 33, 83 e9–10.

McKinney, P. A., Beale, M. D., & Kellner, C. H. 1998. Electroconvulsive therapy in a patient with a cerebellar meningioma. *J ECT*, 14, 49–52.

Mehta, V., Mueller, P. S., Gonzalez-Arriaza, H. L., Pankatraz, V. S., & Rummans, T. A. 2004. Safety of electroconvulsive therapy in patients receiving long-term warfarin therapy. *Mayo Clinic proceedings*. 79, 1396–401.

Montgomery, S. A., & Asberg, M. 1979. A new depression scale designed to be sensitive to change. *Br J Psychiatry*, 134, 382–9.

Mukherjee, S., Sackeim, H. A., & Schnur, D. B. 1994. Electroconvulsive therapy of acute manic episodes: a review of 50 years' experience. *Am J Psychiatry*, 151, 169–76.

Petrides, G., & Fink, M. 1996. Atrial fibrillation, anticoagulation, and electroconvulsive therapy. *Convuls Ther*, 12, 91–8.

Pettinati, H. M., Stephens, S. M., Willis, K. M., & Robin, S. E. 1990. Evidence for less improvement in depression in patients taking benzodiazepines during unilateral ECT. *Am J Psych*, 147, 1029–35.

Popeo, D., & Kellner, C. H. 2009. ECT for Parkinson's disease. *Med Hypotheses*, 73, 468–9.

Pritchett, J. T., Bernstein, H. J., & Kellner, C. H. 1993. Combined ECT and antidepressant drug therapy. *Convuls Ther*, 9, 256–61.

Raskin, D. E. 1984. Cardiac irritability, tricyclic antidepressants, and electroconvulsive therapy. *J Clin Psychopharmacology*, 4, 237–8.

Rasmussen, K., & Abrams, R. 1991. Treatment of Parkinson's disease with electroconvulsive therapy. *Psychiatr Clin North Am*, 14, 925–33.

Rasmussen, K. G., Ryan, D. A., & Mueller, P. S. 2006. Blood glucose before and after ECT treatments in Type 2 diabetic patients. *J ECT*, 22, 124–6.

Rasmussen, K. G., & Zorumski, C. F. 1993. Electroconvulsive therapy in patients taking theophylline. *J Clin Psychiatry*, 54, 427–31.

Rubner, P., Koppi, S., & Conco, A. 2009. Frequency of and rationales for the combined use of electroconvulsive therapy and antiepileptic drugs in Austria and the literature. *World J Biol Psychiatry*, 10, 836–45.

Rush, A. J., Trivedi, M. H., Ibrahim, H. M., et al. 2003. The 16-Item Quick Inventory of Depressive Symptomatology (QIDS), clinician rating (QIDS-C), and self-report (QIDS-SR): a psychometric evaluation in patients with chronic major depression. *Biol Psychiatry*, 54, 573–83.

Sackeim, H. A., Decina, P., Prohovnik, I., Malitz, S., & Resor, S. R. 1983. Anticonvulsant and antidepressant properties of electroconvulsive therapy: a proposed mechanism of action. *Biolo psychiatry*, 18, 1301–10.

Sackeim, H. A., Dillingham, E. M., Prudic, J., et al. 2009. Effect of concomitant pharmacotherapy on electroconvulsive therapy outcomes: short-term efficacy and adverse effects. *Arch Gen Psychiatry*, 66, 729–37.

Schaerf, F. W., Miller, R. R., Lipsey, J. R., & McPherson, R. W. 1989. ECT for major depression in four patients infected with human immunodeficiency virus. *Am J Psychiatry*, 146, 782–4.

Schak, K. M., Mueller, P. S., Barnes, R. D., & Rasmussen, K. G. 2008. The safety of ECT in patients with chronic obstructive pulmonary disease. *Psychosomatics*, 49, 208–11.

Schnur, D. B., Mukherjee, S., Silver, J., Degreef, G., & Lee, C. 1989. Electroconvulsive therapy in the treatment of episodic aggressive dyscontrol in psychotic patients. *Convuls Ther*, 5, 353–61.

Sienaert, P., & Peuskens, J. 2007. Anticonvulsants during electroconvulsive therapy: review and recommendations. *J ECT*, 23, 120–3.

Small, J. G., Klapper, M. H., Kellams, J. J., et al. 1988. Electroconvulsive treatment compared with lithium in the management of manic states. *Arch Gen Psychiatry*, 45, 727–32.

Steingard, R., Khan, A., Gonzalez, A., & Herzog, D. B. 1992. Neuroleptic malignant syndrome: review of experience with children and adolescents. *J Child Adolesc Psychopharmacol*, 2, 183–98.

Stromgren, L. S. 1997. ECT in acute delirium and related clinical states. *Convuls Ther*, 13, 10–7.

Stromgren, L. S., Dahl, J., Fjeldborg, N., & Thomsen, A. 1980. Factors influencing seizure duration and number of seizures applied in unilateral electroconvulsive therapy. Anaesthetics and benzodiazepines. *Acta psychiatrica Scandinavica*, 62, 158–65.

Tancer, M. E., & Evans, D. L. 1989. Electroconvulsive Therapy in Geriatric Patients Undergoing Anticoagulation Therapy. *Convuls Ther*, 5, 102–9.

Tess, A. V., & Smetana, G. W. 2009. Medical evaluation of patients undergoing electroconvulsive therapy. *N Engl J Med*, 360, 1437–44.

Trollor, J. N., & Sachdev, P. S. 1999. Electroconvulsive treatment of neuroleptic malignant syndrome: a review and report of cases. *Australian and New Zealand J psychiatry*, 33, 650–9.

van den Broek, W. W., Birkenhäger, T. K., Mulder, P. G., Bruijn, J. A., & Moleman, P. 2006. Imipramine is effective in preventing relapse in electroconvulsive therapy-responsive depressed inpatients with prior pharmacotherapy treatment failure: a randomized, placebo-controlled trial. *J Clin Psychiatry*, 67, 263–8.

Virupaksha, H. S., Shashidhara, B., Thirthalli, J., Kumar, C. N., & Gangadhar, B. N. 2010. Comparison of electroconvulsive therapy (ECT) with or without anti-epileptic drugs in bipolar disorder. *J Affect Disord*, 127, 66–70.

Weiner, R. D., Whanger, A. D., Erwin, C. W., & Wilson, W. P. 1980. Prolonged confusional state and EEG seizure activity following concurrent ECT and lithium use. *Am J Psychiatry*, 137, 1452–3.

Zielinski, R. J., Roose, S. P., Devanand, D. P., Woodring, S., & Sackeim, H. A. 1993. Cardiovascular complications of ECT in depressed patients with cardiac disease. *Am J Psychiatry*, 150, 904–9.

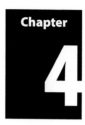

Electroconvulsive Therapy (ECT): Technique

Electrode Placement

There are three commonly used electrode placements in current ECT practice, (bilateral (BL), also known as bitemporal (BT), right unilateral (RUL) and bifrontal (BF)), although the role of bifrontal placement remains to be fully established (Kellner et al., 2010a; Kellner et al., 2010b) We believe that in many cases the decision about which electrode placement to use should be made in collaboration with the patient, after a discussion of the likely advantages and disadvantages of each. In clinical practice, it should be relatively easy to decide whether to use bilateral or unilateral electrode placement. The decision should be based primarily on the severity and urgency of the patient's condition. Bilateral electroconvulsive therapy (ECT) may act more rapidly or completely than right unilateral ECT, but bilateral ECT will have greater cognitive side effects.

Bilateral ECT

Once the decision to proceed with ECT has been made, bilateral ECT should be considered for patients who are judged to be most seriously ill. For depressed patients, indicators of such severity include acute suicidality, poor nutritional status, and severe agitation or psychosis. Some experts suggest that mania should be treated with bilateral ECT (Small et al., 1985). Certainly, bilateral ECT should be considered for patients with severe mania whose extent of psychomotor agitation places them at risk for dehydration and physical exhaustion. Catatonia, in any diagnostic category, is generally considered an indication for bilateral ECT. Although severity of depression must be judged individually for each patient, some general guidelines may be helpful. If a standardized rating scale is used, a score in the upper ranges of the scale may help to confirm the severity of illness. For example, a Hamilton Rating Scale for Depression (HRSD) rating score of 30 or greater (Hamilton, 1960) might favor the use of bilateral electrode placement. Weight loss of greater than 10% of

Brain Stimulation in Psychiatry: ECT, DBS, TMS, and Other Modalities, Charles H. Kellner. Published by Cambridge University Press. © Charles H. Kellner, 2012.

body weight or suicidal preoccupation requiring constant observation might also favor the use of bilateral ECT. Patients who want to be assured of receiving the most powerful and effective form of treatment may express a preference for bilateral over unilateral ECT. Finally, patients with severe medical conditions that might increase the risks of repeated anesthesia sessions should be considered for bilateral electrode placement, because it is most reliably effective and typically has more rapid therapeutic effects, minimizing the number of anesthesia inductions.

Right Unilateral ECT

Unilateral electrode placement should be used for the majority of patients who do not fall into the above category, "most seriously ill." In general, these patients will still be very seriously depressed, but without potentially life-threatening complications of the illness. If the patient fails to respond after 4 to 6 unilateral ECT treatments at adequate stimulus dose, then a switch to bilateral ECT should be strongly considered (Abrams, 2002). Individuals with particular concerns about cognitive impairment, such as those with cognitively demanding jobs, should receive unilateral ECT unless a clear indication for bilateral ECT is present. Those with preexisting cognitive impairment, such as dementia, who have less cognitive reserve should preferably be treated with unilateral electrode placement.

Left-Handedness

Left-handed patients who are being considered for right unilateral ECT pose an interesting problem. Because language function is predominantly located in the left hemisphere in approximately 98% of right-handed people and in 70–90% of left-handed people (Bryden, 1982), it is reasonable to begin unilateral ECT on the right side, even in left-handed patients. If the patient experiences unusually severe confusion or memory impairment after the first few treatments, consideration should be given to switching to left unilateral electrode placement. A simple test of hemispheric dominance can be done, comparing the time elapsed following an ECT treatment until the patient can name simple objects (American Psychiatric Association, 2001; Pratt et al., 1971). It should also be remembered that another option is switching to bilateral electrode placement, with the expectation that efficacy will be enhanced and that cognitive side effects probably will not be increased (Lapidus and Kellner, 2011).

Bifrontal ECT

Bifrontal (BF) electrode has become widely used because it is believed to combine the efficacy of BT placement, with a cognitive effect profile similar to that of RUL placement. Several moderate-sized studies support these contentions (Letemendia et al., 1993; Bailine et al., 2000) while a recently published larger study by the Consortium for Research in Electroconvulsive Therapy (CORE) group failed to confirm these advantages (Kellner et al., 2010a). Technically, BF placement is the easiest to use because there is no hair to interfere with the placement of electrodes. We believe that it is likely that BF placement is more similar to BT than RUL in both efficacy and cognitive effects. Given the smaller evidence base supporting its use, it is difficult to recommend it as the placement of choice; however, it is certainly a viable option. Future studies may help clarify its optimal place in treatment technique.

Location of Electrodes

Although many different electrode sites have been used in the past, in modern ECT, almost all practitioners use three standard placements. For bilateral ECT, the electrode positions are symmetrically located on either side of the forehead just above the midpoint of a line running from the outer canthus of the eye to the external auditory meatus. If a circular metal electrode is used and its inferior edge is placed on this line, the center of the electrode will be approximately 1 inch above the line. As noted above, this placement is synonymously referred to as either "bilateral," "bitemporal," or sometimes, "bifrontotemporal" (Figure 4.1).

For right unilateral ECT, the right electrode position is the same as for bilateral ECT, and the other (vertex, or bregma) electrode is placed with the left (medial) electrode edge touching a line that runs down the middle of the skull at its intersection with a perpendicular line connecting the two external auditory canals (Figure 4.2). If the left edge of the electrode disc is at this vertex position,

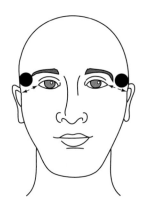
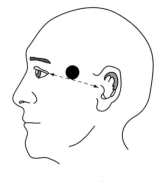

Figure 4.1. Bilateral electrode placement.

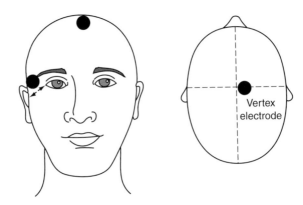

Figure 4.2. Right unilateral electrode placement.

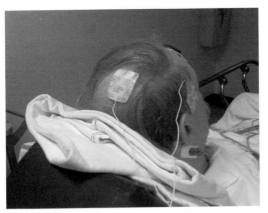

Figure 4.3. Patient set up for right unilateral ECT (d'Elia placement), using disposable, adhesive stimulus pads.

the center of the electrode will be approximately 1 inch to the right of the vertex. This configuration is known as the d'Elia placement, after the psychiatrist who developed it (d'Elia, 1970) (Figure 4.3). For BF electrode placement, the location of the electrodes is on the forehead, with the center of the electrode placed approximately 5 cm above the outer canthus of the eye. Given the anatomical differences between peoples' foreheads, the exact location will differ slightly between patients. (Figure 4.4)

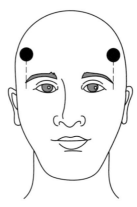

Figure 4.4. Bifrontal electrode placement.

It is important to remember that optimal electrode placement will allow for the greatest distance between the two electrodes while staying as closely as possible at the anatomical landmark outlined above. The technique of preparing the electrode sites is covered in the section below, "Electrode Site Preparation."

Stimulus Dosing

Choosing the appropriate strength of the stimulus (the electrical "dose") has become an important part of contemporary ECT practice. Nowadays, the practitioner needs to make decisions about both stimulus characteristics (primarily pulse width) and intensity (primarily expressed in terms of charge.) Obviously, the stimulus has to be sufficient to induce a generalized seizure – the therapeutic goal of ECT – but beyond that, the situation becomes more complex. Some generalized ECT seizures, if induced with a stimulus very close to seizure threshold (particularly with right-sided electrode placement), may not be maximally therapeutic; thus, in certain situations, it may be advantageous to give stimuli that are several times greater than the seizure threshold (see below). On the other hand, stimuli that are far in excess of the seizure threshold (particularly with bilateral electrode placement) may contribute to excess cognitive impairment. Several options are available to the ECT practitioner for attempting to deal with this clinical dilemma. We will review the available methods below, including (1) stimulus dose titration, (2) age-based dosing, (3) fixed high-dose therapy, and (4) dosing estimates based on patient characteristics (e.g., age, sex). The issue of the use of ultrabrief pulse stimuli will be discussed in a separate section (see below).

Stimulus Dose Titration

First, let us define *seizure threshold*. Quite simply, seizure threshold is the minimum amount of electrical stimulus needed to induce a seizure. But "amount" in terms of what? *Charge* is probably the best unit of measurement to describe the stimulus, although, unless the stimulus characteristics are fully described (frequency, pulse width, duration, and current), even *charge* does not tell the whole story. Some ECT devices describe their output in terms of joules (J), with the assumption that a patient's impedance will be close to the standard value of 220 ohms. It should be remembered, however, that even though such devices indicate the "energy" setting in joules, they are constant-current devices, and, therefore, this setting will be an approximation, and you are really setting the exact amount of charge to be delivered. Thus, patient seizure threshold may be expressed in terms of either charge or joules, but more commonly charge. With dose titration, a patient's seizure threshold is determined at the first ECT session. This "method of limits" involves starting at low stimulus levels and administering a series of increasingly strong stimuli until a seizure occurs (Beale et al., 1994b; Coffey et al., 1995; Sackeim et al., 1993). After the delivery of each stimulus, one observes the patient and the EEG recording on the ECT device to determine if a seizure has been elicited. If both a robust motor and EEG seizure are observed, then the patent's seizure threshold has been found. If no motor or EEG seizure are detected, continue to observe the patient and run the EEG recording paper for at least 20 seconds (this is to not miss a possibly delayed-onset seizure). In the case of an equivocal EEG seizure and no observed motor seizure, we recommend that one conclude that no seizure has occurred. In the case of a well-developed EEG seizure and no motor seizure, the field is divided as to what to do. We recommend re-stimulating at the next step in the titration algorithm, which usually then results in both a robust motor as well as EEG, seizure. Of course, if there is an explanation for the absence of the motor seizure, for example, if the cuff was not properly inflated on the ankle, then re-stimulation may not be advisable. When re-stimulating, the ECT device paper strip is stopped, impedance is re-checked, the bite block is again positioned, the ECT device is set to the next (higher) stimulus in the algorithm and the stimulus is delivered.

To some extent, the choice of stimulus settings is arbitrary and specific to the ECT device being used. The general principle is quite simple, however, and should be universally applicable: start with a setting near the lowest output of the device and increase that by 50–100% for each subsequent stimulus. Remember to consult the instruction manual of your ECT device to help in establishing the specific sequence you will use in your practice.

Almost all patients will have had a seizure by the fourth setting in your dose titration sequence. For the rare situations in which a patient does not have a seizure with the fourth stimulus, you will have to decide whether it is safe to deliver a fifth stimulus at the maximal setting on the ECT device. This decision will depend on several factors, including the patient's medical condition, the type and amount of anesthesia given, and the urgency of the psychiatric illness. Your overriding concerns should be (1) patient safety and (2) eliciting a seizure. We agree with the American Psychiatric Association (American Psychiatric Association, 2001) statement: "in general, patients should not leave the ECT suite failing to have had a seizure." Some clinicians believe that multiple stimuli are associated with greater side effects, such as headache, nausea, and hypertension.

Some patients require modification of the general principles outlined above. Most important, young patients will probably require a very low stimulus charge. Unless there are extenuating circumstances, adolescents and young adults (<30 years old) should be stimulated first at the lowest setting of the device.

At the other end of the spectrum, very elderly patients or patients who are being treated while continuing to take anticonvulsant medication(s) may need a higher stimulus charge than the standard sequence above. For example, for an 80-year-old man being treated with phenytoin, the dose may be titrated starting at approximately 100 mC, rather than 25 mC or lower.

What should you do with the seizure threshold information obtained at the first ECT session? The general principle is that you should use the information to make a rational choice of stimulus dose for subsequent treatments. Let us take the following four examples of young and old patients with right unilateral and bilateral electrode placement to illustrate:

Example 1. *Young patient, right unilateral electrode placement*

A 32-year-old man had no seizure at 25 mC but had a 45-second seizure at 50 mC. Thus, his seizure threshold is somewhere between these two stimuli, but we do not know it more precisely than this. In practice, we arbitrarily select the higher number as the probable seizure threshold. Thus, we assume the seizure threshold is 50 mC.

Now, because there is reasonable evidence that charge should exceed seizure threshold several-fold with right unilateral electrode placement (say, by a multiple of 6 (Sackeim et al., 2009), we would select a stimulus 6 times higher than the seizure threshold for the second treatment session. Thus, 50 mC × 6 = 300 mC

What about the stimulus dose in treatments 3 and beyond? Most practitioners would continue treatments at the same stimulus dose unless: (1) the patient is not improving as expected, (2) the seizures become "inadequate" (i.e., missed, very short, or of very low EEG amplitude), or (3) the patient is having excessive cognitive effects. For situations 1 and 2, the stimulus dose could be adjusted up by increments of 25–50%. For situation 3, the stimulus dose could be lowered, or other steps taken to decrease the cognitive effects of the treatment (e.g., increasing the time interval between treatments).

Example 2. *Young patient, bilateral electrode placement*

A 28-year-old woman has a 60-second seizure at the initial stimulus of 25 mC; thus, we know that her seizure threshold is below 25 mC, but we do not know it more precisely than that. (The situation is one in which the standard dose titration settings have proved imperfect, because, ideally, a patient should not seize at the first setting, so that a lower limit of the threshold can be found.) We arbitrarily assume that her seizure threshold is 25 mC. At the second treatment, we recommend that she be treated at 50 mC, because, with bilateral electrode placement, the stimulus need only exceed the seizure threshold by a moderate amount (e.g., 1.5–2 X seizure threshold).

Example 3. *Older patient, right unilateral electrode placement*

A 76-year-old woman has no seizure at 50 mC but has a 38-second seizure at 100 mC. Thus, we know that her seizure threshold is between 50 mC and 100 mC, but we do not know it more precisely than this. We arbitrarily assume her seizure threshold is 100 mC. For treatment 2, we would multiply by a factor of 6, which places us above the range of the device. Thus, for treatment 2 and subsequent treatments, we would treat this patient at a setting near the top of the device, between 375 and 500 mC. The concept is that with right unilateral electrode placement, the stimulus dose should be several multiples of the seizure threshold.

Example 4. *Older patient, bilateral electrode placement*

An 82-year-old man has no seizure at 50 mC, 100 mC, or 200 mC but has a 42-second seizure at 400 mC. Thus, we know that his seizure threshold is between 200 mC and 400 mC, but we do not know it more precisely than this. We arbitrarily assume his seizure threshold is 400 mC. For treatment 2, we recommend treating at 400 mC, because it is likely that this stimulus is actually a reasonable amount above his seizure threshold, given the wide spacing between the levels in the dose titration algorithm used. The stimulus dose could be adjusted up or down at subsequent treatments, based on seizure adequacy and cognitive effects of the treatment course.

Age-Based Dosing

An alternative to dose titration is to make an educated guess about the patient's seizure threshold and then choose a stimulus charge that is likely to be sufficiently above that threshold to produce effective antidepressant results, while minimizing cognitive effects. Because seizure threshold increases with age, the most commonly recommended system has been to select a dose based on the patient's age. For example, Abrams and Swartz (2009), in the Thymatron ECT Instruction Manual, suggest setting the percentage of energy at the patient's age (for bilateral electrode placements). A similar system could be used with the joule units on a MECTA device. Although this method results in satisfactory treatments for most patients, there are some patients for whom the dose will probably be substantially above their seizure threshold, and excessive cognitive impairment can result. Using bilateral electrode placement, this method, on average, results in a stimulus dose 250% above threshold (Beale et al., 1994b). In addition, this age-based dosing does not take into account the major differences between dosing requirements in bilateral and right unilateral electrode placement. Petrides and Fink (1996) recommended a modification of age-based dosing that they call the one-half age method: setting the charge on the ECT device at the percentage of energy one-half the patient's age. This method decreases the likelihood of administering grossly suprathreshold stimuli (Petrides et al., 2009).

Fixed High-Dose Therapy

A third method of stimulus dosing involves giving a fixed high charge to all patients without determination of their seizure threshold (Abrams et al., 1991). Many practitioners believe this strategy exposes the patient to unnecessarily high stimulus doses, which may lead to more cognitive impairment. However, this method is useful in severely ill patients in whom a rapid, definitive response is needed. For example, treating a catatonic or agitated manic patient at 80–100% stimulus charge for the duration of the ECT course may provide a more rapid and sustained response than near-threshold dosing.

Dosing Estimates Based on Patient Characteristics

Some practitioners use stimulus dosing charts to determine the appropriate dose for a given patient. These charts are based on patient characteristics known to be associated with seizure threshold. These include the patient's age, sex, laterality of electrode placement, and other variables (see the ECT device manufacturer instruction manuals). This method, however, provides only an educated guess about the patient's true threshold and is therefore less accurate than empirical seizure threshold determination.

Ultrabrief Pulse Stimuli

Ultrabrief pulse stimuli are becoming more commonly used in contemporary ECT. By arbitrary convention, "ultrabrief" is defined as a pulsewidth less than 0.5 ms; brief pulse is defined as a pulsewidth between 0.5–2.0 ms. Both the MECTA and Thymatron ECT devices are capable of delivering ultrabrief or brief pulsewidth stimuli. There is no reason to believe that 0.5 ms is a magical dividing line between brief and ultrabrief stimuli; rather it is more likely that there is a continuum of effects, with narrower pulsewidths possibly associated with lesser cognitive effects.

There is increasing evidence that the use of ultrabrief pulse stimuli is associated with diminished cognitive impairment, compared with standard brief pulse stimuli (Sienaert et al., 2010). While the emerging data also support the clinical efficacy of ultrabrief pulse stimuli, it remains to be seen if the antidepressant efficacy and speed of response are, in fact, comparable to standard brief pulse stimuli.

Several reports document the use of ultrabrief stimuli with RUL ECT. At least one study documents the efficacy of ultrabrief stimuli with bifrontal ECT (Sienaert et al., 2009). There is no reason to doubt the efficacy of ultrabrief stimuli with bilateral electrode placement, despite one report with a small sample suggesting it is ineffective; it is more likely that this result was anomalous (Sackeim et al., 2008).

Seizure thresholds are markedly lower with ultrabrief pulse stimuli and dose titration algorithms and subsequent dosing strategies may need to be adjusted accordingly.

Electrode Site Preparation

The preparation of the scalp for stimulus delivery and electroencephalogram (EEG) monitoring is a crucial part of the ECT procedure. The reader should supplement the instructions for site preparation reviewed here with the particular recommendations of the ECT device manufacturer. To verify proper skin contact, a self-test procedure should be a standard part of the preparation for ECT stimulus delivery.

EEG Recording Electrodes

A minimum of two channel (4 leads) EEG recording should be standard procedure for all ECT. One lead is placed on the left side of the forehead, one on the right side of the forehead, one behind the left ear, over the mastoid bone, and one behind the right ear. This lead placement, referred to as left and right frontomastoid, allows monitoring of seizure activity in the both hemispheres; this is appropriate for both bilateral and right unilateral ECT.

The frontal lead should be placed 1 inch above the eyebrow in the mid-pupillary line. The mastoid lead should be placed behind the left ear, as high on the mastoid process as allowed by the patient's hairline. This location helps to avoid artifact from the left carotid artery (see Figure 4.5). Both EEG sites should be cleaned with alcohol and then dried. Disposable, self-adhesive electrodes are then applied; make sure that they adhere tightly.

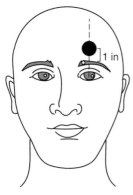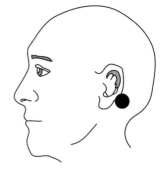

Frontal EEG lead placement   Mastoid EEG lead placement

Figure 4.5. Electroencephalogram (EEG) placement.

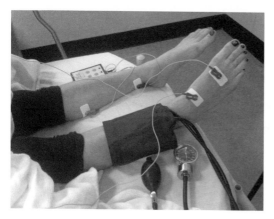

Figure 4.6. Patient set up showing electromyogram and blood pressure cuff on right foot, nerve stimulator on left calf.

Electromyogram (EMG) Recording Electrodes

One ECT device (the Thymatron) uses a 2-lead, single-channel EMG to measure motor seizure activity. The EMG electrodes should be placed approximately 3 inches apart on the dorsum of the right foot (see Figure 4.6). The sites are cleaned with alcohol and allowed to dry, and the same disposable, stick-on electrodes used for the EEG are applied. The MECTA ECT device uses an optical motion sensor wrapped around the patient's finger or toe to detect the motor seizure, in a manner analogous to the EMG.

Stimulus Site Preparation

The preparation of the stimulus sites is crucial for safe and effective ECT (see previous section, "Electrode Placement," for an anatomical guide to stimulus electrode location). The practitioner should refer to the instruction manual of his or her ECT device for further details of site preparation.

Right Unilateral Considerations

For site preparation in right unilateral ECT, attention must first be given to parting the hair at the vertex. This part must provide sufficient scalp exposure for good electrode-to-scalp contact. As noted below, a metal handheld electrode will often be necessary for the vertex site, rather than a disposable stick-on. Other aspects of site preparation are identical for unilateral and bilateral ECT.

Metal Stimulus Electrodes

When using metal electrodes, both scalp sites are first cleansed with a gauze pad soaked in saline. Conductive gel is then applied to the stimulus electrodes and, when manual electrode paddles are used, the electrodes are placed on the stimulus site after the patient is anesthetized; sufficiently firm pressure must be maintained to allow good skin contact throughout the delivery of the stimulus. This sequence may be somewhat different when a headband is used to hold electrodes in place. Refer to the ECT device instruction manual for further direction in the use of the headband, if this method is to be used. The vertex metal electrode is hand held with a paddle, whereas the frontotemporal electrode may be either hand held or held in place with a headband.

Disposable, Stick-on Electrodes

Many practitioners choose to use disposable stimulus electrodes, which adhere to the patient's scalp. When these electrodes are used, the site should be moistened with saline, followed by the application of a few drops of "pre-tack" solution. Additional "pre-tack" can be directly applied to the adhesive side of the electrode before application. The practitioner should then press the electrodes into place, with special attention to good skin adherence across the entire surface. The vertex electrode, for unilateral ECT, will often require a hand held cupped paddle over the site to maintain adequate contact.

See Figure 4.7 for a summary of the placement of recording and stimulus electrodes.

The Self-Test Procedure

Following placement of the stimulus electrodes and before delivery of the stimulus, adequate integrity of the electrical circuit should be documented by a self-test procedure. This procedure involves the passage of a small amount of

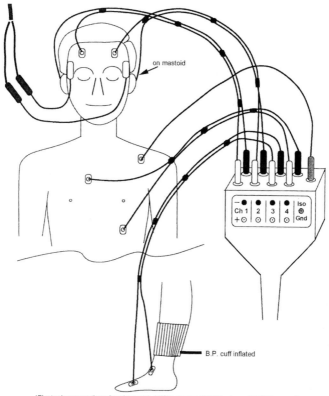

4 channel setup---2 EEG, 1 EMG, 1 ECG channel *

on mastoid

−● ● ● ● | Iso
Ch 1 | 2 | 3 | 4 | ⊕
+⊙ | ⊙ | ⊙ | ⊙ | Gnd

B.P. cuff inflated

*Electrode connections for channel 1, 2 EEG, channel 3 EMG, channel 4 ECG recording

Figure 4.7. Patient set-up showing recording (EEG, EMG, EKG) and stimulus electrodes used on a contemporary ECT device. (Used with permission from Somatics, LLC.)

current (below the patient's sensory threshold) to measure the impedance of the circuit. *The cause of an abnormal impedance value should be fully evaluated and corrected before stimulus delivery.*

High Impedance

An abnormally high impedance (e.g., greater than 2800 ohms) represents a failure of smooth current flow through the circuit. Common causes include improper skin preparation and/or inadequate skin-to-electrode contact and inadequate connection of the stimulus cable to the electrodes or the ECT device.

Low Impedance

An impedance that is too low (e.g., less than 100 ohms) is very rare, and indicates an accessory pathway for current flow. This shunt may be due to communicating conductive gel between the electrodes or conduction occurring through some other substance, such as hair gel or excessive perspiration. A short circuit in the stimulus cable is another possible cause. *In the case of either too low or too high impedance, the cause of the problem should be remedied before delivery of the stimulus.*

Physiological Monitoring

Vital signs, blood oxygen saturation, electrocardiogram (ECG), EEG, and EMG are all continuously monitored during ECT. In addition, a nerve stimulator should be used to monitor the effects of succinylcholine.

Vital Signs

Pulse and blood pressure should be followed at close intervals before, during, and after ECT. An automated blood pressure cuff is ideal for these purposes and is strongly recommended. A baseline pressure and pulse should be recorded before any medication is given. If pretreatment antihypertensive agents (e.g., esmolol or labetalol) are given, 15 minutes should be allowed for the agent(s) to work and a repeat set of vital signs should be recorded. Poststimulus vital signs should be recorded every 35 minutes until a stable baseline is achieved (usually approximately 10 minutes). More frequent or longer monitoring schedules can be used for patients for whom there are particular concerns about cardiovascular management.

Pulse Oximetry

It is now standard anesthesia practice to monitor blood oxygen saturation by pulse oximetry continuously before and during ECT and in the immediate post-ECT recovery period. This simple, noninvasive monitoring procedure provides the practitioner with crucial information about the patient's respiratory status. Most patients should have an oxygen saturation at, or near, 100% during most of the procedure.

The pulse oximeter probe can be placed on a finger, toe, or earlobe. It should be on a limb without a blood pressure cuff, because inflation of the cuff interrupts the probe's functioning.

Electrocardiogram

The ECG is monitored using standard leads. The tracing is continuously displayed on an oscilloscope screen and may also be printed out. The ECG can be printed out by the ECT device itself.

Electroencephalogram

EEG monitoring is a crucial part of modern ECT practice. It enables the practitioner to confirm that a cerebral seizure has occurred and that the seizure has ended in a timely manner. This is a crucial point and bears repeating: *EEG monitoring is most important for determining that the seizure is over.*

Although the 4-lead, two-channel EEG used in most ECT cannot provide the sophisticated information of a standard 16-lead EEG, it is adequate for the requirements of ECT.

The now-standard left and right frontomastoid recording sites fulfill the important criteria of adequate interelectrode distance and, with right unilateral electrode placement, the ability to know that the seizure has generalized to the left hemisphere (Figure 4.5). Furthermore, these sites eliminate the possible problem of one side canceling out the other, as can occur when two frontal (one on either side of the forehead) leads are used for the same channel.

Interpretation of the EEG has been the subject of considerable discussion and controversy in the ECT literature. In practice, it should become a matter of routine for the practitioner to adequately record and interpret the EEG. Adequate recording is ensured by careful attention to recording site location and preparation, setting of amplifier gain, and exclusion of artifact. (See previous section, "Electrode Site Preparation," and section below, "Treatment Procedure.") Interpretation of the ECT EEG is largely a matter of common sense: the seizure ends when the EEG goes flat. Most of the time, this determination is a very simple one. Sometimes, however (e.g., when the EEG amplitude decreases gradually rather than abruptly), it is difficult to determine exactly when the seizure ends (although after a few seconds it will become clear that the seizure is over). In rare instances, the EEG, despite one's best efforts, is uninterpretable. In such cases, the practitioner will need to rely on clinical signs (resumption of spontaneous breathing, return to baseline heart rate) to know that the seizure is over. See Figures 4.8 and 4.9 for sample tracings from modern ECT devices.

A major part of EEG interpretation is being able to distinguish artifact from true cerebral activity. Examples of the most commonly encountered artifacts are shown in Figure 4.10.

Electromyogram

Monitoring EMG is a way to provide a backup measurement (and hard-copy tracing) of the length of the motor seizure. Currently, one ECT device, the

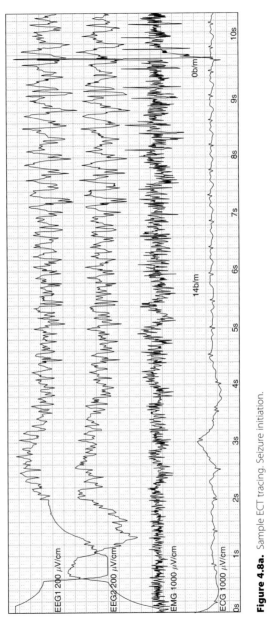

Figure 4.8a. Sample ECT tracing. Seizure initiation.

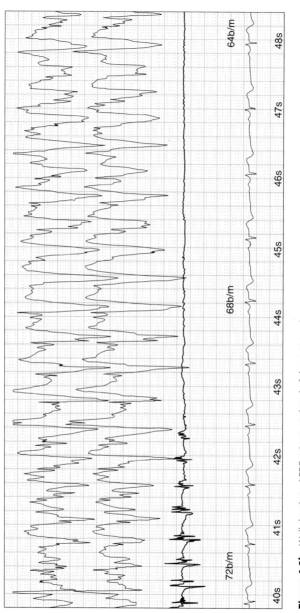

Figure 4.8b. Well developed EEG seizure and end of the motor seizure.

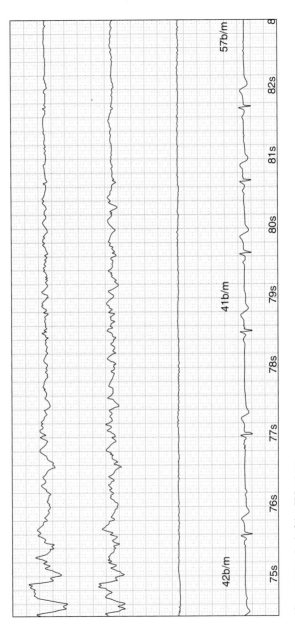

Figure 4.8c. End of the EEG seizure.

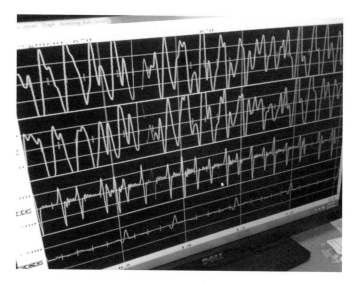

Figure 4.9. Computer monitor showing seizure in progress. Top two lines are left and right frontomastoid EEG, third line is electromyogram (EMG), bottom line is electrocardiogram (ECG).

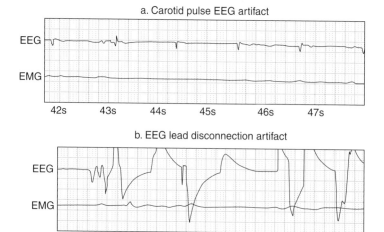

Figure 4.10. Recording artifacts.

Thymatron, provides a channel specifically for EMG monitoring. (The MECTA has an analogous feature, the Optical Motion Sensor, which serves the same function.) Two extra-long leads are attached to the dorsum of the right foot (see Figure 4.6). The tracing is interpreted in the same way as is the EEG. When the EMG tracing goes flat, the motor seizure is over; the length of the seizure is noted from the timing marks on the recording paper. See Figure 4.8 for an example of EMG patterns during each phase of the ECT seizure.

EMG recordings may also be subject to artifact. Occasionally, the impulse from the nerve stimulator may cause a recurrent blip on the EMG tracing. More commonly, moving the patient or the EMG leads during recording also produces artifact.

Nerve Stimulator

A peripheral nerve stimulator is used to assess the muscle relaxant effect of succinylcholine (Kellner, 2011). Several anatomical sites can be used: in the arm, along the radial or ulnar nerves; in the leg, along the posterior tibial nerve; or on the dorsum of the foot. We recommend placement of the nerve stimulator along the posterior tibial nerve, as pictured in Figure 4.6. Using a site on the leg rather than on the arm allows more accurate assessment of when the effects of succinylcholine are maximal, because the drug works in a rostrocaudal progression. We also recommend a nerve stimulator with an automatic setting such that the progressive decrement in response can be easily observed. Alternatively, one can simply monitor the plantar reflexes or repeatedly check the tone of the limbs. Generally, it takes approximately 1 minute for the succinylcholine to have maximal effect in a young patient, and about 2 minutes in many older patients (see section "Muscular Relaxation").

Anesthetics and Muscular Relaxation

A professional trained in anesthesia is a required member of the ECT treatment team. The anesthesia experience should be brief and uncomplicated for most patients; the primary goals are patient safety and comfort.

Anesthetics

Brief, light general anesthesia is used during ECT to achieve amnesia, absence of pain for the procedure, and allow the use of succinylcholine for muscular relaxation (see Table 4.1 for a comparison of various agents used in ECT anesthesia).

Methohexital

Methohexital has become the standard anesthetic for ECT because it has rapid onset, has brief duration, and causes minimal postanesthesia confusion. It is

Table 4.1. ECT Anesthetics

Agent	Usual Dose (mg/kg)	Relative Anticonvulsant Effect	Comments
Methohexital	0.75–1.0	1	Standard agent for ECT; rapid recovery; pain on injection
Thiopental	2.0–5.0	2	Cardiovascular depression
Propofol	1.0–2.5	3	Pain on injection; may shorten seizures
Etomidate	0.2–0.3	0	Myoclonus; adrenal suppression; less cardiovascular depression
Ketamine	0.5–2.0	−1 (proconvulsant)	Hypertension; tachycardia; hallucinations
Alfentanil (adjunctive)	0.010–0.015	1	Increased duration of apnea; reduced hypertension and tachycardia; reduced hypnotic dose
Remifentanil (adjunctive)	0.001–0.008	−1 (proconvulsant)	Reduced hypnotic dose; attenuated hemodynamic response

less anticonvulsant than other barbiturates. Dosing is typically 0.75–1.0 mg/kg body weight, given as an intravenous bolus of a 1% solution (i.e., 10 mg/mL). The minimum required dose is often lower in elderly patients. Methohexital is a local irritant and often burns upon intravenous injection; however, it causes only brief discomfort, because unconsciousness rapidly ensues.

Thiopental

Thiopental has a longer duration of action and is more anticonvulsant than methohexital. The early suggestion that thiopental produced more cardiac arrhythmias than methohexital (Pitts et al., 1965) is controversial and has not been born out in subsequent usage.

Propofol

Propofol has become the second most commonly used induction agent in ECT. It has the advantages of causing less hypertension and tachycardia than methohexital as well as less post-ictal agitation. Patients may experience a "smoother" anesthesia experience with this agent. However, it is markedly more anticonvulsant than other induction agents and is associated with shorter seizures and increased seizure thresholds. Because of these anticonvulsant properties, it may be the agent of choice for ECT in children and adolescents (Bailine et al., 2003), many of whom may have prolonged seizures early in their treatment course.

Etomidate

Etomidate is a good alternative anesthetic with acceptably low anticonvulsant properties. It has less negative effect on cardiac contractility than methohexital and may be preferable in patients with heart failure. Myoclonic jerks are often seen during the drug's onset of action. Repeated doses have been reported to cause adrenocortical insufficiency, although this is probably an uncommon occurrence.

Ultrashort-acting Narcotics

Recently, ultrashort-acting narcotics, such as alfentanil and remifentanil, have been used in combination with propofol, methohexital, or etomidate to induce anesthesia for ECT. In general, using an adjunctive narcotic reduces hypnotic dose, increases seizure duration, and attenuates hemodynamic responses to ECT (Recart et al., 2003).

Ketamine

Ketamine is interesting as an alternative ECT anesthetic because of both its proconvulsant and intrinsic antidepressant properties (Berman et al., 2000). It is an NMDA antagonist compound related to phencyclidine (PCP) and can induce psychotic symptoms. Practitioners have used it without encountering such problems (Rasmussen et al., 1996). There is accumulating evidence that its use in ECT can accelerate antidepressant response and possibly reduce cognitive adverse effects (Okamoto et al., 2010). It is associated with a higher incidence of hypertension during the procedure.

Muscular Relaxation

Muscular relaxation is used during ECT to eliminate musculoskeletal injury and to aid in airway management. Complete paralysis is not required except in cases of severe osteoporosis or unstable vertebral column.

Succinylcholine

The preferred neuromuscular blocking agent for ECT is succinylcholine, primarily because of its rapid onset and brief duration of action. Succinylcholine dosing is usually 0.75–1.0 mg/kg of lean body mass. Higher doses (up to 1.3 mg/kg) may be used when complete paralysis is required. Succinylcholine is typically given as a rapid intravenous bolus of a solution of 20 mg/mL, which should be refrigerated until just before use. Succinylcholine should only be given after the patient is unconscious. A patent airway should be present before succinylcholine dosing, because the drug paralyzes the diaphragm.

Assessment of Muscular Relaxation

The adequacy of muscular relaxation may be measured by a peripheral nerve stimulator and by the loss of tone and reflexes in a distal extremity. Because succinylcholine is a depolarizing agent, muscle fasciculations occur as the drug reaches the neuromuscular junction. The disappearance of fasciculations is a marker that full circulation of the drug has occurred. Elderly patients often have a longer latency of action than younger patients (Beale et al., 1994a). Waiting approximately 60 seconds following injection of succinylcholine in young patients, and 120 seconds in geriatric patients is usually adequate.

Fasciculation Muscle Pain

Especially after the first treatment, diffuse musculoskeletal pain due to fasciculations may occur. The pain is responsive to simple analgesics (e.g., nonsteroidal anti-inflammatory drugs) and typically lessens with subsequent treatments. If the pain persists after subsequent treatments, fasciculations may be attenuated by pretreatment with a small dose of a nondepolarizing muscle relaxant.

Cuff Technique

Before succinylcholine injection, a blood pressure cuff on the right ankle should be inflated above the patient's systolic pressure to prevent succinylcholine access to that foot. This procedure allows focal observation of the motor seizure. The right side of the body is used to document seizure generalization to the contralateral hemisphere in the case of right unilateral ECT, and, of course, is also suitable for use with bilateral placements. In situations where the right leg cannot be used (e.g., severe edema, skin infection) the left foot or a forearm may be used.

Nondepolarizing Muscle Relaxants

Nondepolarizing muscle relaxants (e.g., mivacurium, rocuronium, cisatracurium, and others) have a slower onset and a longer duration of action than succinylcholine. They are used in ECT for special situations, including pseudocholinesterase deficiency (usually a familial disorder) and risk of excessive potassium release with succinylcholine, as is seen in cases of severe burns, massive tissue trauma, or severe spasticity or paralysis (American Psychiatric Association, 2001). Reversal agents (e.g., neostigmine) and an anticholinergic agent (e.g., glycopyrrolate) will also need to be given.

Anticholinergic Agents

The routine use of anticholinergic premedication to prevent vagal bradyarrhythmias during ECT is controversial. Preexisting cardiac conduction delay, the use of β-adrenergic antagonists, and dose titration procedures, which may involve multiple subconvulsive stimuli, all argue for anticholinergics to be used. Arguments against their use include the induction of increased heart rate and blood pressure, constipation, urinary retention, and potential amnestic effects. A reasonable practice would be to administer an anticholinergic agent at the first treatment in a course if a dose titration procedure is being done, and then omit it at subsequent treatments.

Glycopyrrolate

Glycopyrrolate (a peripheral anticholinergic that does not cross the blood-brain barrier) is given in doses of 0.2–0.4 mg intravenously at the time of the procedure. Note that glycopyrrolate is almost always given for the sole purpose of preventing bradycardia. When the additional effect of decreasing secretions is desired, it must be given approximately 10 minutes before the procedure.

Atropine

Atropine is a more potent vagolytic agent than glycopyrrolate. Atropine doses range from 0.4 to 1.0 mg intravenously at the time of the procedure.

Oxygenation

The patient should receive supplemental oxygen, 100%, by means of mask, throughout the procedure. It is prudent to oxygenate just before the procedure, especially in patients with a history of myocardial ischemia. For all patients, as soon as unconsciousness is produced by the barbiturate, positive-pressure ventilation at 15–20 breaths/minute should begin and continue until spontaneous respiration resumes. Oxygen saturation should be maintained at or near 100% throughout the procedure. Vigorous hyperventilation should be given for patients in whom a longer seizure is desired. This can be started immediately after the succinylcholine is injected, and continued (with a break for the insertion of the bite block and stimulus delivery) until the desired seizure length is achieved.

Airway Management and NPO Status

Airway management

The anesthetist should carefully evaluate the patient's mouth and airway before ECT for any potential problem areas. Loose teeth should be documented and may need extraction before the procedure. Solitary teeth, loose teeth, or asymmetrical bite bearing by teeth may require evaluation by a dentist before ECT. For some patients, the insertion of an oral airway may facilitate ventilation.

Bite Block

When the patient is ready for stimulus delivery, the oxygen mask should be removed while a protective foam or rubber bite block is inserted into the mouth. The bite block should be inserted so as to push the tongue inferiorly and posteriorly into the mouth, behind the teeth. The bite block should then be placed against the upper teeth, and the lower teeth and jaw should be held up to firmly meet the bottom surface of the bite block. The lips should be pulled safely over the bite block. The chin should be pushed upward with firm pressure during the stimulus. This action absorbs the jaw flexion that occurs as a result of the direct effects of the stimulus on, and the poor succinylcholine blockade of these muscles. The bite block is usually removed after stimulus delivery. For some patients it may be left in place to facilitate ventilation by the anesthetist. It may also be left in place if delivery of a second stimulus is being considered.

Nothing by Mouth (NPO)

Because of concern about aspiration of gastric contents during anesthesia, patients are to have nothing by mouth (NPO) for 8 hours before the procedure. When a patient has taken small amounts of liquids or clear liquids the morning of ECT, the anesthesiologist should be consulted and consideration should be given to treating the patient after a short (e.g., 2-hour) waiting period.

Intubation

Patients very rarely require intubation for ECT. In certain situations (e.g., the third trimester of pregnancy, severe gastroparesis, or severe gastroesophageal reflux), the anesthesiologist may elect to intubate the patient. In the large majority of cases of gastroesophageal reflux, pretreatment with a histamine-2 H_2-blocker taken with a sip of water approximately 2 hours before ECT, should be sufficient aspiration prophylaxis.

Cardiovascular Agents

It is helpful to conceptualize two categories of cardiovascular drugs for ECT patients:

1) Those that are taken regularly to treat chronic hypertension, arrhythmias, ischemia, or other cardiac conditions, and
2) Those that are given adjunctively just before or during the ECT procedure to blunt the hypertensive, tachycardic response to the seizure

In general, a patient's regular cardiovascular medication should be continued during a course of ECT, including antihypertensives, digoxin, and antiarrhythmics. Exceptions to this rule are diuretics on the mornings of treatment (because a patient should not have a full bladder at the time of treatment) and reserpine at any point during an ECT course (because of the risk of hypotension). Fortunately, reserpine is no longer in routine use. Medications can be given by mouth with a sip of water 1–2 hours before ECT. The most important adjunctive cardioactive agents are discussed below.

The main goals of the use of adjunctive agents are to reduce the risk of myocardial ischemia (a possible result of the increased oxygen demand associated with tachycardia) and to reduce the risk of systemic hypertension. It should be kept in mind that, although it seems intuitively obvious that careful control of heart rate and blood pressure would be beneficial, little data exist comparing cardiovascular morbidity in ECT done with and without adjunctive antihypertensive agents.

β-Blockers

Esmolol

Esmolol is an ultrashort-acting drug (half-life 9 minutes) that decreases heart rate but has relatively less effect on blood pressure. Its rapid onset and short duration of action make it a nearly ideal agent for use in ECT. Typical bolus doses are 10–50 mg, but higher doses are sometimes used.

Labetalol

Labetalol is a short-acting combined alpha- and beta-blocker (half-life 5 hours) that decreases both heart rate and blood pressure. Typical bolus doses range from 5 to 20 mg. Because its duration of action is longer than that of esmolol, there is a risk of inducing hypotension in the post-ECT period.

β-blockers should be used with caution in patients with asthma, cardiac conduction delay, or heart failure.

Other Antihypertensives

While far less commonly used than beta-blockers, several other antihypertensive agents can be used effectively in conjunction with ECT at the time of the procedure. These include calcium channel blockers (e.g., nicardipine), hydralazine, and nitroglycerin.

Calcium Channel Blockers

Nicardepine (Cardene) has replaced sublingual nitrates and, to some extent, other calcium channel blockers to control blood pressure during ECT because it can be given IV and titrated more deliberately than sublingual medications (Zhang et al., 2005). Diltiazem (Cardizem) (Wajima et al., 2001) and verapamil (Isoptin) (Wajima et al., 2002) are two other calcium channel blockers that are available in intravenous preparations.

Hydralazine

Hydralazine is an older "classic" agent that works well to reduce blood pressure but may cause tachycardia. Typical doses are 5–40 mg. Because the average maximal vasodilation occurs after 10–80 minutes, hypotension in the post-ECT period could be a risk.

Nitroglycerin

Nitroglycerin is an extremely helpful agent used to decrease the risk of myocardial ischemia and to reduce blood pressure. It is available as a transdermal paste, a sublingual tablet or spray, or intravenous infusion. While we previously recommended transdermal or sublingual use before the procedure, we now limit our recommendations mainly to the use of intravenous nitroglycerin to control hypertension in at-risk patients during and shortly after the procedure. Transdermal nitroglycerin may occasionally be used after ECT for its longer duration of action.

When used intravenously, nitroglycerin provides nearly immediate lowering of blood pressure and can be titrated for effective blood pressure control.

Lidocaine

This potent antiarrhythmic is also a potent anticonvulsant and thus is problematic to use in conjunction with ECT. When serious ectopy or ventricular arrhythmias appear during or after the seizure, a bolus dose of 50–100 mg may be given. If possible, to prevent interference with the seizure, the injection of lidocaine should be delayed until the motor seizure ends.

It should be emphasized that decisions about the use of potent cardioactive agents should be made in concert with the anesthesia staff. Exactly which patients to treat or pretreat remains a matter of clinical judgment and some controversy. Patients with a history of angina or myocardial infarction should be most carefully assessed, and steps taken to avoid excessive oxygen demand on the heart. Elderly patients with hypertension may be best treated with small doses of labetalol or esmolol. The risks of side effects of these drugs (mainly hypotension) need to be balanced against the potential risks of the treatment itself.

Often, we do not use these agents at the first treatment, preferring merely to observe whether clinically significant rises in heart rate or blood pressure occur. If these changes are deemed problematic, medication can be given immediately, then prophylactic use of antihypertensives can be instituted for subsequent treatments. This would typically consist of giving 5 or 10 mg IV labetalol several minutes before the procedure.

Missed, Short, and Prolonged Seizures

The vast majority of ECT seizures last between 25 and 70 seconds. Some weak evidence suggests that very short seizures (less than 15–20 seconds) may be less therapeutic than longer seizures, particularly if they are elicited by near-threshold stimuli. Some stronger evidence suggests that very long seizures (more than 2–3 minutes) may be associated with more cognitive impairment than shorter seizures, particularly if they are elicited by stimuli far in excess of seizure threshold.

The issue of how to define seizure length requires comment. Because both the motor seizure and the EEG seizure are measured, which one to use to determine seizure length is quite important, albeit arbitrary (Howsepian, 2011). We will define seizures as follows:

- A missed seizure is one in which no motor activity develops following delivery of the stimulus.
- A short seizure is one in which the motor manifestations of the seizure last <15 seconds.
- A prolonged seizure is one in which motor or EEG seizure activity persists >180 seconds.

Interestingly, we choose the motor seizure to define a short seizure and the EEG seizure to determine a prolonged seizure. This is a conservative position, because it tends to favor restimulation at the short end of the spectrum and definitive intervention at the long end of the spectrum. It should be remembered that the EEG seizure typically lasts longer (e.g., 10–30% longer) than the motor seizure and that one occasionally sees the development of an EEG seizure without a motor seizure, but only very rarely a motor seizure without an EEG seizure (and when this occurs, it is probably due to a technical failure to record the EEG properly). It is important that the ECT practitioner be prepared to deal with these three situations.

Missed Seizures

Most missed seizures occur during the stimulus dose titration procedure done at the first treatment (see the previous section, "Stimulus Dosing"). If dose titration is carried out, and stimuli are appropriately chosen at successive treatments, missed seizures (other than those seen during dose titration) will be uncommon. When they do occur, it will probably be toward the end of a treatment course in an elderly patient with a very high seizure threshold or in a patient taking anticonvulsants. A missed seizure should prompt a routine sequence of steps. These are discussed below.

Missed Seizure During Dose Titration

See the subsection, "Stimulus Dose Titration."

Missed Seizure in the Middle of an ECT Course

Follow the steps below, in order.

1. Be sure to observe the patient long enough (approximately 20 seconds) to ascertain that a delayed seizure does not occur. (The seizure may be delayed when the stimulus is just at threshold.)

2. Continue to hyperventilate the patient while checking the printed output on the ECT device to be sure that the desired stimulus was actually given. (Premature release of the stimulus delivery button is one cause of missed seizures in the middle of an ECT course.)

3. Check the electrical connections to the stimulus electrodes for tightness and continuity. Check the stimulus electrode delivery sites for adequate preparation, repeating any of the site preparation steps deemed necessary (see previous section, "Electrode Site Preparation").

4. After a 20- to 30-second wait, repeat the impedance check, reinsert the bite block, and restimulate the patient at a higher stimulus intensity. How much higher will depend on the level of the previous (subconvulsive) stimulus. (Note that this can be determined by the use of a stimulus dosing algorithm, examples of which appear in the ECT device manufacturers' instruction manuals.) If, for example, a patient has a missed seizure at a stimulus dose of 285 millicoulombs [mC]), it would be reasonable to restimulate at a 50% higher stimulus, approximately 425 mC. If this procedure is also ineffective, it is reasonable to restimulate at the highest setting on the ECT device. If a determination of a high initial seizure threshold has been made for a given patient, and that patient reaches the maximum setting on the ECT device through incremental dosing and then misses a seizure, it is reasonable to give a period of vigorous hyperventilation and then a second maximal stimulus. If this second maximal stimulus is also ineffective, we recommend no further stimuli at that treatment session.

5. If the patient is to have additional treatments, thoroughly review the factors likely to have contributed to the missed seizure. These factors include (1) excessive anesthetic dose, (2) concurrent anticonvulsant drug(s), (3) an older patient late in the course of treatment, and (4) technical factors (premature release of the stimulus button, poor electrical connections) unrelated to the patient's seizure threshold. Appropriate corrective measures (e.g., lowering the dose of the anesthetic or the anticonvulsant) can then be carried out before the next treatment.

Short Seizures

Seizures lasting less than 15 seconds are a fairly common occurrence, particularly late in the course of treatment of an elderly patient. Short motor seizures are also more common with the use of ultrabrief stimuli. Because short seizures may be less effective, it is reasonable to attempt to increase seizure length into the "acceptable" range. *However, some patients may do well despite short seizures, and in such cases, no technical modifications are required.*

A motor seizure of less than 15 seconds should prompt the following routine steps:

1. Decide whether to restimulate. Restimulation should ordinarily be attempted, unless there is some unusual overriding concern (e.g., development of a cardiovascular complication such as arrhythmia or severe hypertension) or the patient is doing well clinically and their typical seizure length is very short.
2. Hyperventilate the patient vigorously for approximately 60 seconds.
3. Reinsert the bite block, do a repeat impedance check, and restimulate at an approximately 50% higher stimulus level, or the maximum setting on the ECT device (if the previous stimulus was in the upper range of the ECT device).
4. If the patient is to have additional treatments, thoroughly review the factors likely to have contributed to the short seizure. Most commonly, these are (1) excessive anesthetic dose, (2) a concurrent anticonvulsant (either a "true" anticonvulsant, such as phenytoin [Dilantin] or carbamazepine, or another drug with anticonvulsant properties, such as a benzodiazepine or lidocaine), (3) lack of good hyperventilation, and 4) inadequate electrical stimulus dose.

It should be emphasized that some patients (particularly elderly patients near the end of a course of treatment) have short seizures regardless of modifications in technique. Most of these patients do very well, and drastic measures to increase seizure length are clearly unwarranted.

There is evidence that for a given charge, prolonging the stimulus duration can lead to more efficient seizure elicitation (Sackeim et al., 1994). Contemporary ECT devices offer several different stimulus program options that allow for longer stimulus durations. This type of adjustment may be used as an option when patients have short seizures.

Another strategy commonly used in the past for seizure prolongation was the intravenous administration of caffeine (available as caffeine sodium benzoate), an adenosine antagonist, 5 minutes before ECT (Coffey et al., 1987). Cardiac-rate-controlling agents may be required with caffeine, and caution must be exercised when using caffeine in patients with a history of cardiac ischemia or arrhythmia. The dose of caffeine for this usage ranges from 125 to 2,000 mg, starting with lower doses and increasing at subsequent treatments as needed. There is debate over whether caffeine lowers the seizure threshold or prolongs seizure duration or both (McCall et al., 1993). While some practitioners continue to use caffeine as an adjunctive medication in ECT, we no longer recommend it, given the uncertainty of the risk-benefit ratio.

Prolonged Seizures

Prolonged seizures are of greater concern than short seizures because of their potential to lead to adverse effects, particularly cognitive impairment. Therefore, it is crucial to be vigilant for seizures lasting more than 2 or 3 minutes. The report of the APA Task Force on ECT (American Psychiatric Association, 2001) states, "a prolonged seizure is one that is longer than 3 minutes by motor or EEG manifestations. Some practitioners use a more stringent definition of 2 minutes" (p. 171). We begin to become concerned when a seizure lasts more than 120 seconds, and we generally begin to intervene by 130–140 seconds. Seizure prolongation should be determined by the EEG, because the most common occurrence is the continuation of EEG seizure activity after the motor seizure has ended. Non-convulsive status epilepticus refers to the condition in which the cerebral seizure persists despite the lack of motor manifestations. Of course, if the motor seizure is also prolonged, or if for some reason the EEG cannot be recorded or interpreted, the motor seizure is obviously used to determine seizure prolongation.

Once the decision to terminate a prolonged seizure is made, the following steps should be taken:

1. Administer an anticonvulsant drug. We recommend giving approximately 50% of the dose of the anesthetic drug used (except in cases in which ketamine was used). For example, if a patient had been given 60 mg of methohexital for induction, now a 30-mg intravenous bolus should be given. An alternative would be to give an intravenous benzodiazepine (e.g., 1–2 mg IV lorazepam [Ativan] or midazolam [Versed]).
2. Continue to oxygenate (but not hyperventilate) and carefully monitor the cardiovascular status of the patient while watching the EEG for cessation of epileptiform activity.
3. If after 1–2 minutes the seizure is still ongoing, repeat the medication given above.
4. Continue pharmacological interventions along with full medical support of the patient until seizure activity is ended.

A prolonged seizure should prompt a thorough review of the factors likely to have contributed to its occurrence, including (1) concurrent administration of a proconvulsant medication (e.g., theophylline), (2) metabolic disturbance (e.g., hyponatremia), and (3) structural brain disease. It should be remembered that some young patients have long seizures at the lowest stimulus settings on the ECT device, particularly in the first several treatments. Such patients may routinely require administration of additional doses of the anesthetic agent to end their seizures. Propofol may be a particularly good choice of induction agent in these patients (Bailine et al., 2003).

Treatment Procedure

Outlined below is a list of steps required for a typical ECT procedure:

(Note that some details of the sequence may need to be modified for the particular requirements of the ECT device you are using; remember to consult the instruction manual of your device for details.)

Table 4.2. Pre-ECT Orders

– NPO after midnight

– Void on call to ECT

– Take cardiac and anti-gastric reflux medications with sip of water approximately 2 hours before ECT (if prescribed)

Note. NPO = nothing by mouth.

1. Confirm that the patient has had nothing to eat or drink that morning, has taken the appropriate premedications, and has signed informed consent (Table 4.2). Then have him or her lie down on the treatment bed.
2. Start the intravenous line. Although it may seem obvious, it cannot be overstated that a well-functioning intravenous line is the cornerstone of safe ECT. This does not necessarily suggest that the intravenous line must be a large-bore catheter attached to an intravenous bag; a small butterfly or catheter, if carefully inserted and well secured in place, works just as well. Typical sites are the dorsum of the hand, the forearm, and the antecubital region. The larger the vein, the less likely it is that the injection of methohexital will be painful. For this reason, an antecubital vein is the preferred site.
3. Attach the blood pressure cuff and the ECG leads.
4. Record vital signs.
5. Place a second blood pressure cuff on the right ankle.
6. Prepare the EEG recording sites and stimulus electrode sites as per the ECT device instruction manual.
7. Select the electrical stimulus dose on the ECT device.
8. Attach the EEG, ECG, and EMG electrodes of the ECT device. Apply stimulus electrodes if using stick-on type.
9. Perform the tap test to check EEG and EMG sensitivity. The amplifier sensitivity should be adjusted so that a finger tap on the electrode produces a large positive and negative deflection of the tracing, with a quiet baseline between taps (see Figure 4.11).
10. Administer methohexital, 1 mg/kg intravenously.
11. Apply stimulus electrodes if using hand held type.
12. Perform impedance self-test on the ECT device.
13. Begin assisted ventilation with 100% oxygen.
14. Inflate the blood pressure cuff on the right ankle
15. Ensure that the patient is unconscious, then administer succinylcholine, 0.75–1.0 mg/kg intravenously.
16. Start nerve stimulator to assess muscular relaxation. Observe for decrement and eventual disappearance of response.

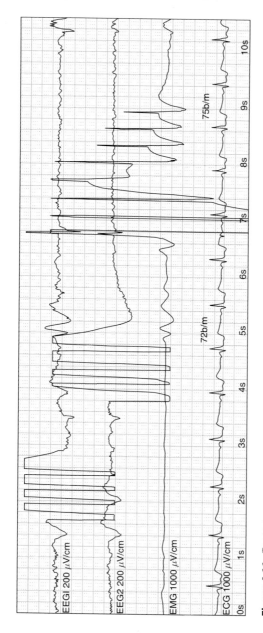

Figure 4.11. Tap test.

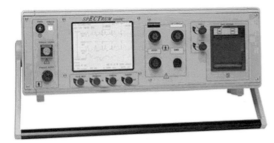

Figure 4.12. The MECTA spECTrum 5000Q. Used with the manufacturer's permission.

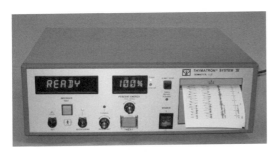

Figure 4.13. The Thymatron System IV device. Used with permission from Somatics, LLC.

17. Simultaneously observe for fasciculations. Wait until they subside in the calves and toes.

18. Insert the bite block, making sure that the tongue is pushed inferiorly and posteriorly in the mouth and that the chin is held firmly against the bite block.

19. Deliver the electrical stimulus.

20. Remove the bite block and resume ventilation. Observe the motor and the EEG seizures, noting the duration of both.

21. When the motor seizure ends, deflate the blood pressure cuff on the right ankle.

22. Allow the patient to awaken in as unstimulating an environment as possible.

23. Monitor vital signs in the treatment and then recovery areas.

References

Abrams, R. 2002. *Electroconvulsive Therapy.* New York: Oxford University Press.

Abrams, R. & Swartz, C. M. 2009. *Thymatron System IV Instruction Manual*, Fourteenth Edition, July 2009. Somatics, LLC.

Abrams, R., Swartz, C. M., & Vedak, C. 1991. Antidepressant effects of high-dose right unilateral electroconvulsive therapy. *Arch Gen Psychiatry*, **48**, 746–8.

American Psychiatric Association. 2001. *Task Force on Electroconvulsive Therapy. The Practice of Electroconvulsive Therapy: Recommendations for Treatment, Training, and Privileging.* Washington, DC: American Psychiatric Association.

Bailine, S. H., Petrides, G., Doft, M., & Lui, G. 2003. Indications for the use of propofol in electroconvulsive therapy. *J ECT*, **19**, 129–32.

Bailine, S. H., Rifkin, A., Kayne, E., et al. 2000. Comparison of bifrontal and bitemporal ECT for major depression. *Am J Psychiatry*, **157**, 121–3.

Beale, M. D., Kellner, C. H., Lemert, R., et al. 1994a. Skeletal muscle relaxation in patients undergoing electroconvulsive therapy. *Anesthesiology*, **80**, 957.

Beale, M. D., Kellner, C. H., Pritchett, J. T., et al. 1994b. Stimulus dose-titration in ECT: a 2-year clinical experience. *Convuls Ther*, **10**, 171–6.

Berman, R. M., Cappiello, A., Anand, A., et al. 2000. Antidepressant effects of ketamine in depressed patients. *Biol Psychiatry*, **47**, 351–4.

Bryden, M. P. 1982. *Laterality: Functional Asymmetry in the Intact Brain.* New York: Academic Press.

Coffey, C. E., Lucke, J., Weiner, R. D., Krystal, A. D., & Aque, M. 1995. Seizure threshold in electroconvulsive therapy: I. Initial seizure threshold. *Biol Psychiatry*, **37**, 713–20.

Coffey, C. E., Weiner, R. D., Hinkle, P. E., et al. 1987. Augmentation of ECT seizures with caffeine. *Biol Psychiatry*, **22**, 637–49.

d'Elia, G. 1970. Unilateral electroconvulsive therapy. *Acta Psychiatr Scand Suppl*, **215**, 1–98.

Hamilton, M. 1960. A rating scale for depression. *J Neurol Neurosurg Psychiatry*, **23**, 56–62.

Howsepian, A. A. 2011. On describing "seizure length" in electroconvulsive therapy. *J ECT*, **27**, 93–4; author reply 94.

Kellner, C. H. 2011. Muscle relaxation in electroconvulsive therapy. *J ECT*, **27**, 93; author reply 93.

Kellner, C. H., Knapp, R., Husain, M. M., et al. 2010a. Bifrontal, bitemporal and right unilateral electrode placement in ECT: randomised trial. *Br J Psychiatry*, **196**, 226–34.

Kellner, C. H., Tobias, K. G., & Wiegand, J. 2010b. Electrode placement in electroconvulsive therapy (ECT): a review of the literature. *J ECT*, **26**, 175–80.

Lapidus, K. A., & Kellner, C. H. 2011. When to switch from unilateral to bilateral electroconvulsive therapy. *J ECT*, **27**, 244–6.

Letemendia, F. J., Delva, N. J., Rodenburg, M., et al. 1993. Therapeutic advantage of bifrontal electrode placement in ECT. *Psychol Med*, **23**, 349–60.

McCall, W. V., Reid, S., Rosenquist, P., Foreman, A., & Kiesow-Webb, N. 1993. A reappraisal of the role of caffeine in ECT. *Am J Psychiatry*, **150**, 1543–5.

Okamoto, N., Nakai, T., Sakamoto, K., et al. 2010. Rapid antidepressant effect of ketamine anesthesia during electroconvulsive therapy of treatment-resistant depression: comparing ketamine and propofol anesthesia. *J ECT*, **26**, 223–7.

Petrides, G., Braga, R. J., Fink, M., et al. 2009. Seizure threshold in a large sample: implications for stimulus dosing strategies in bilateral electroconvulsive therapy: a report from CORE. *J ECT*, **25**, 232–7.

Petrides, G., & Fink, M. 1996. The "half-age" stimulation strategy for ECT dosing. *Convuls Ther*, **12**, 138–46.

Pitts, F. N., Desmarais, G. M., Stewart, W., & Schaberg, K. 1965. Induction of anesthesia with methohexital and thiopental in electroconvulsive therapy. The effect on the electrocardiogram and clinical observations in 500 consecutive treatments with each agent. *N Engl J Med* **273**, 353–60.

Pratt, R. T., Warrington, E. K., & Halliday, A. M. 1971. Unilateral ECT as a test for cerebral dominance, with a strategy for treating left-handers. *Br J Psychiatry*, **119**, 79–83.

Rasmussen, K. G., Jarvis, M. R., & Zorumski, C. F. 1996. Ketamine anesthesia in electroconvulsive therapy. *Convuls Ther*, **12**, 217–23.

Sackeim, H. A., Dillingham, E. M., Prudic, J., et al. 2009. Effect of concomitant pharmacotherapy on electroconvulsive therapy outcomes: short-term efficacy and adverse effects. *Arch Gen Psychiatry*, **66**, 729–37.

Sackeim, H. A., Long, J., Luber, B., et al. 1994. Physical properties and quantification of the ECT stimulus: I. Basic principles. *Convuls Ther*, **10**, 93–123.

Sackeim, H. A., Prudic, J., Devanand, D. P., et al. 1993. Effects of stimulus intensity and electrode placement on the efficacy and cognitive effects of electroconvulsive therapy. *N Engl J Med*, **328**, 839–46.

Sackeim, H. A., Prudic, J., Nobler, M. S., et al. 2008. Effects of pulse width and electrode placement on the efficacy and cognitive effects of electroconvulsive therapy. *Brain Stimul*, **1**, 71–83.

Sienaert, P., Vansteelandt, K., Demyttenaere, K., & Peuskens, J. 2009. Randomized comparison of ultra-brief bifrontal and unilateral electroconvulsive therapy for major depression: clinical efficacy. *J Affect Disord*, **116**, 106–12.

Sienaert, P., Vansteelandt, K., Demyttenaere, K., & Peuskens, J. 2010. Randomized comparison of ultra-brief bifrontal and unilateral electroconvulsive therapy for major depression: cognitive side-effects. *J Affect Disord*, **122**, 60–7.

Small, J. G., Small, I. F., Milstein, V., Kellams, J. J., Klapper, M. H. 1985. Manic symptoms: an indication for bilateral ECT. *Biol Psychiatry*, **20**, 125–34.

Wajima, Z., Yoshikawa, T., Ogura, A., et al. 2001. The effects of diltiazem on hemodynamics and seizure duration during electroconvulsive therapy. *Anesth Analg*, **92**, 1327–30.

Wajima, Z., Yoshikawa, T., Ogura, A., et al. 2002. Intravenous verapamil blunts hyperdynamic responses during electroconvulsive therapy without altering seizure activity. *Anesth Analg*, **95**, 400–2, table of contents.

Zhang, Y., White, P. F., Thornton, L., Perdue, L., Downing, M. 2005. The use of nicardipine for electroconvulsive therapy: a dose-ranging study. *Anesth Analg*, **100**, 378–81.

Chapter 5

Electroconvulsive Therapy (ECT): Treatment Course

Treatment Schedule

Number of Treatments

There is no standard number of electroconvulsive therapy (ECT) treatments in a course and a patient cannot be told in advance exactly how many treatments he/she will need to remit. Most patients will require between 6 and 12 treatments, but some will require as few as 3 or 4 and some as many as 20. There are reports of rare complete recoveries after 1 or 2 treatments (Kobeissi et al., 2011; Thomas and Kellner, 2003).

The patient should be treated until one of the following therapeutic end points is achieved:

1. Full recovery.
2. A plateau in improvement is reached, and no further gains have been seen after the last two treatments.

A treatment course should be interrupted in the case of any of the following events:

1. Unacceptably serious cognitive effects occur.
2. A medical complication occurs that renders further treatment unsafe at the time.
3. Consent is withdrawn.
4. Additionally, some practitioners suggest that when a bipolar depressed patient switches into hypomania, a quite rare event (Bailine et al., 2010), the treatment course be stopped. Others argue that, because ECT also treats mania, the course should be continued until the patient is euthymic. We believe continuing the course is appropriate in most situations.

Diagnosis

There are few convincing data showing that a particular diagnosis requires more or fewer treatments in a course. The exception to this is the evidence that

Brain Stimulation in Psychiatry: ECT, DBS, TMS, and Other Modalities, Charles H. Kellner. Published by Cambridge University Press. © Charles H. Kellner, 2012.

bipolar depression responds slightly more quickly than unipolar depression (Sienaert et al., 2009). Some practitioners believe, on the basis of clinical experience, that patients with schizophrenia require longer treatment courses and also that some patients with catatonia require prolonged courses for full recovery. In most cases, application of the previously mentioned two criteria for therapeutic end points will allow for rational, flexible decision making about how long to continue ECT.

Treatment Frequency

Routine practice in the United States is to give ECT three times a week on a Monday-Wednesday-Friday schedule. This schedule was probably originally designed around the schedule of the treating physician, but it works very well to balance good speed of recovery with some between-treatment time for recovery of memory function (Stromgren, 1990).

Elderly patients, or those for whom there are particular concerns about cognitive adverse effects, may be treated twice a week (e.g., Monday and Friday). Recovery from depression may be expected to be slower (Lerer et al., 1995). A twice-a-week ECT schedule is routinely used in the United Kingdom and other countries.

Some practitioners have suggested that right unilateral ECT, because it causes less cognitive impairment than bilateral ECT, may be given more frequently than three times a week (4 or even 5 times a week) (Abrams, 1967). Ultrabrief pulse right unilateral ECT, with its particularly benign cognitive side effect profile, may provide opportunities for more flexible treatment scheduling.

Very seriously ill patients, including those who are severely manic, catatonic, or malnourished, can be given daily bilateral ECT until some evidence of recovery is seen.

Clinical Monitoring

To be able to make informed decisions about when to stop or continue treatment, close clinical monitoring of the patient is required. This monitoring should be done by daily interviews (or, at a minimum, before each treatment), paying attention to the patient's report of mood, energy level, reduction in psychotic symptoms (if present), and memory function. Reports by hospital staff (for inpatients) or family (for outpatients) of the patient's behavior and ability to function are also essential.

Information gathered from patient, staff, and family should be supplemented by objective rating scales. Many excellent depression rating scales are available, including the Hamilton Rating Scale for Depression (HRSD or "HAM-D") (Hamilton, 1960). This scale should be given before ECT is begun, at least once weekly during the course of ECT, and at the completion

Table 5.1. Strategies to Consider if Substantial Cognitive Dysfunction Develops

– Switch from bilateral to unilateral electrode placement

– Decrease treatment frequency (from three times weekly to twice or once weekly)

– Decrease stimulus dose

– Review concurrent medications for contribution to cognitive dysfunction

of the ECT course – preferably by the same person – and the score should be recorded in the patient's medical record.

Objective measures of cognitive functioning are also important to follow during a course of ECT. Again, many test instruments are available and acceptable, including the Mini-Mental State Exam (MMSE) (Folstein et al., 1975). Although it provides only a crude estimate of cognitive functioning, this test has the advantage of being simple and quick to administer. It should be given before the ECT course is begun and then weekly during the course of ECT, preferably on non-treatment days, or in the morning, before the next treatment. Significant declines (e.g., from 27 to 19) should prompt more detailed clinical assessment of the patient and consideration of stopping or interrupting the treatment course. The MoCA is another brief assessment tool that can be used for following global cognitive function during a course of ECT (Nasreddine et al., 2005). If severe cognitive dysfunction develops, other strategies may also be helpful (Table 5.1).

It will come as a pleasant surprise to the beginning ECT practitioner that many patients show improvement, rather than deterioration, in their MMSE scores, because the cognitive impairments of depression ("depressive pseudo-dementia") resolve with ECT.

Continuation/Maintenance ECT

Affective disorders are increasingly recognized as recurrent illnesses. Whereas decades ago, most patients would remit with a course of ECT and remain well for many years without maintenance therapy, this, unfortunately, is no longer the case for many patients. The concept of "treatment resistance" has been offered as an explanation for this phenomenon, but in truth, we do not fully understand this apparent change in the natural history of mood disorders (Sackeim et al., 1990). Choices for modalities of continuation/maintenance treatment are medications or ECT, singly or in combination. Medications may be given as monotherapy, but more commonly as combinations. When given as continuation/maintenance therapy after remission of the index episode, medication (either monotherapy or combination therapy) clearly reduces relapse rates of unipolar depression (Frank et al., 1990; Sackeim et al., 2001). The

CORE continuation ECT vs. pharmacotherapy study demonstrated that continuation ECT, given without medications, was as effective in preventing relapse after successful ECT as the combination pharmacotherapy lithium and nortriptyline (Kellner et al., 2006). Earlier studies found continuation/maintenance ECT to reduce hospitalization rates in patients with recurrent mood disorders (Petrides et al., 1994).

ECT is unique among psychiatric treatments in that it is typically withdrawn once it has proved effective. The lesson to be learned from the above discussion is that some type of continuation/maintenance therapy (either medication(s) or ECT, or both), is necessary after ECT to maximize the chances of sustained remission. Our practice is to taper most acute ECT courses over a couple of weeks and then to offer continuation (arbitrarily defined as therapy in the 6-month period following the index course of ECT) or maintenance (defined as therapy continuing beyond 6 months after the index course) ECT to patients with a history of relapse on medication following response to ECT. Continuation or maintenance ECT involves single treatments, given at increasing intervals, tailored to deliver the minimum number of treatments required to maintain remission (Monroe, 1991; Lisanby et al., 2008).

Frequency of Treatments/Electrode Placement

There is no single continuation/maintenance ECT schedule that is applicable to all patients; some degree of individualization and clinical judgment is required. The acute course (3×/week) can be followed by a taper to 2×/week, then weekly for several weeks. The interval between treatments can then be gradually extended, the goal being to determine the maximal interval that results in maintenance of full remission. Most patients will end up on a schedule of a single treatment every 3–6 weeks, although some will require more frequent treatment.

The electrode placement used in continuation/maintenance ECT is typically that which was used in the index course of ECT, although an argument could be made for the use of bilateral electrode placement because single treatments at long intervals are not expected to cause significant cognitive impairment (Kellner et al., 1991).

Inpatient Versus Outpatient Treatment

Most maintenance ECT patients can be treated as outpatients; however, an overnight stay in the hospital is required in some circumstances. These instances include the patient who cannot reliably avoid taking anything by mouth before treatment and the patient who requires close medical management before or after ECT.

For a full review of issues related to ambulatory ECT, the reader should consult a task force report on ambulatory ECT (Fink et al., 1996).

Monitoring During Maintenance ECT

The patient's medical status should be followed closely during maintenance ECT. Laboratory data (e.g., electrolytes and electrocardiography) should be obtained at appropriate intervals. Cognitive status and depressive symptoms should be followed and rated.

Continuation or Maintenance ECT End Point

After 6–12 months of successful continuation or maintenance ECT, a trial of medication and/or psychotherapy as maintenance therapy should be discussed with the patient and his or her family. Some patients with highly recurrent illness will require maintenance ECT for extended periods, and sometimes indefinitely.

References

Abrams, R. 1967. Daily administration of unilateral ECT. *Am J Psychiatry*, **124**, 384–6.

Bailine, S., Fink, M., Knapp, R., et al. 2010. Electroconvulsive therapy is equally effective in unipolar and bipolar depression. *Acta Psychiatr Scand*, **121**, 431–6.

Fink, M., Abrams, R., Bailine, S., & Jaffe, R. 1996. Ambulatory electroconvulsive therapy: report of a task force of the association for convulsive therapy. Association for Convulsive Therapy. *Convuls Ther*, **12**, 42–55.

Folstein, M. F., Folstein, S. E., & McHugh, P. R. 1975. "Mini-mental state". A practical method for grading the cognitive state of patients for the clinician. *J Psychiatric Res*, **12**, 189–98.

Frank, E., Kupper, D. J., Perel, J. M., et al. 1990. Three-year outcomes for maintenance therapies in recurrent depression. *Arch Gen Psychiatry*, **47**, 1093–9.

Hamilton, M. 1960. A rating scale for depression. *J Neurol Neurosurg Psychiatry*, **23**, 56–62.

Kellner, C. H., Burns, C. M., Bernstein, H. J., & Monroe, R. R., Jr. 1991. Electrode placement in maintenance electroconvulsive therapy. *Convuls Ther*, **7**, 61–2.

Kellner, C. H., Knapp, R. G., Petrides, G., et al. 2006. Continuation electroconvulsive therapy vs pharmacotherapy for relapse prevention in major depression: a multisite study from the Consortium for Research in Electroconvulsive Therapy (CORE). *Arch Gen Psychiatry*, **63**, 1337–44.

Kobeissi, J., Aloysi, A., Tobias, K., Popeo, D., & Kellner, C. H. 2011. Resolution of severe suicidality with a single electroconvulsive therapy. *J ECT*, **27**, 86–8.

Lerer, B., Shapira, B., Calev, A., et al. 1995. Antidepressant and cognitive effects of twice- versus three-times-weekly ECT. *Am J Psychiatry*, **152**, 564–70.

Lisanby, S. H., Sampson, S., Husain, M. M., et al. 2008. Toward individualized post-electroconvulsive therapy care: piloting the Symptom-Titrated, Algorithm-Based Longitudinal ECT (STABLE) intervention. *J ECT*, **24**, 179–82.

Monroe, R. R., Jr. 1991. Maintenance electroconvulsive therapy. *Psychiatr Clin North Am*, **14**, 947–60.

Nasreddine, Z. S., Phillips, N. A., Bedirian, V., et al. 2005. The Montreal Cognitive Assessment, MoCA: a brief screening tool for mild cognitive impairment. *J Am Geriatrics Soc*, 53, 695–9.

Petrides, G., Dhossche, D., Fink, M., & Francis, A. 1994. Continuation ECT: relapse prevention in affective disorders. *Convuls Ther*, 10, 189–94.

Sackeim, H. A., Haskett, R. F., Mulsant, B. H., et al. 2001. Continuation pharmacotherapy in the prevention of relapse following electroconvulsive therapy: a randomized controlled trial. *JAMA*, 285, 1299–307.

Sackeim, H. A., Prudic, J., Devanand, D. P., et al. 1990. The impact of medication resistance and continuation pharmacotherapy on relapse following response to electroconvulsive therapy in major depression. *J Clin Psychopharmacol*, 10, 96–104.

Sienaert, P., Vansteelandt, K., Demyttenaere, K., & Peuskens, J. 2009. Ultra-brief pulse ECT in bipolar and unipolar depressive disorder: differences in speed of response. *Bipolar Disord*, 11, 418–24.

Stromgren, L. S. 1990. Frequency of ECT treatments. *Convuls Ther*, 6, 317–8.

Thomas, S. G., & Kellner, C. H. 2003. Remission of major depression and obsessive-compulsive disorder after a single unilateral ECT. *J ECT*, 19, 50–1.

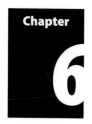

Electroconvulsive Therapy (ECT): Common Adverse Effects

Cognition

The most troublesome and feared adverse effect of electroconvulsive therapy (ECT) is memory loss. In fact, ECT typically causes predictable, largely temporary, memory loss and other cognitive effects that are generally not serious and are very acceptable, given the substantial relief from serious depression that most patients can expect from ECT (Semkovska and McLoughlin, 2010). Modern ECT techniques have markedly reduced the effects on memory for most patients.

An older, detailed review of the effects of ECT on memory function can be found in the *Annals of the New York Academy of Sciences* (Squire, 1986). A more recent, comprehensive reference is the special issue of the *Journal of ECT* on cognition (Loo, 2008). For our purposes, we can summarize ECT's effects on memory and cognition as follows:

ECT affects memory/cognition in three ways. It causes:

1. An acute postictal confusional state,
2. Anterograde memory dysfunction (AMD),
3. Retrograde memory dysfunction (RMD).

Postictal Confusional State

All patients have some degree of confusion and disorientation immediately following ECT. This side effect is more pronounced with bilateral ECT than with right unilateral ECT, and it may be more prolonged in elderly patients. Generally, within a very few minutes of awakening, patients are able to follow simple commands and then begin to speak. Initial disorientation and confusion generally subside within 10–20 minutes and typically are resolved within an hour. With ultrabrief pulse right unilateral ECT, reorientation may occur in several minutes.

Patients must be carefully supervised and monitored by nursing staff during the immediate post-ECT period. A quiet, low-stimulus environment is optimal.

Brain Stimulation in Psychiatry: ECT, DBS, TMS, and Other Modalities, Charles H. Kellner. Published by Cambridge University Press. © Charles H. Kellner, 2012.

Approximately 10% of patients will develop marked agitation and restlessness immediately postictally ("emergence delirium") (Abrams 2002). This is usually easily managed with a short-acting, rapid-onset benzodiazepine such as midazolam (1–4 mg) administered intravenously. If a patient has become agitated at a previous treatment session, at the next session, to prevent the development of agitation, the benzodiazepine may be given as soon as spontaneous respirations resume following the treatment. Patients should be monitored for continuation of spontaneous respirations following administration of benzodiazepines in this setting.

Anterograde Memory Dysfunction

AMD refers to the impaired ability to record new memories after receiving ECT. It can be thought of as disruption of current memory function. Usually this amnesia involves patients' inability to remember things that they have done or were told on the days following ECT. (For example, when you see Ms. Jones at 5:00 P.M. on the ward, she may not remember having spoken with you at 11:00 A.M. that day. Or, in another example, Mr. Smith reports difficulty in remembering where he has left his eyeglasses in the house in the week following ECT.) AMD is worst immediately after ECT and subsides within days or a few weeks. AMD is more severe after a course of bilateral ECT than a course of right unilateral ECT (and probably less with ultrabrief pulse than brief pulse right unilateral) and more severe after a course of ECT (either type) than after a single maintenance treatment.

Retrograde Memory Dysfunction

RMD refers to the forgetting of memories from the pre-ECT period. Because our memories are precious to us and central to our sense of self and individuality, this particular memory effect of ECT is of greatest concern to patients. Fortunately, RMD is almost always limited to the weeks or few months before the start of ECT. The principle of last-in-first-out applies; that is, memories recorded most proximally to the start of ECT are most vulnerable to being lost, and memories recorded in the more remote past are less vulnerable. We make it a practice to tell patients to expect that they will have little recollection of events during the weeks of their ECT course and they may have spotty memory loss for the 3–6 months or so before that. It must be emphasized that there is tremendous variability in this regard: most patients report that the amount of memory loss is acceptable, given the benefit of recovery from severe depression, and that as more time elapses, they are less bothered by any residual memory gaps. We encourage family members to remind patients repeatedly of events that occurred in the pre-ECT interval so that any gaps can be filled in. Occasionally, patients report that they do not want to be reminded of events from the period during which they were severely depressed. This behavior should not be confused with the erroneous notion that ECT works by causing patients to forget how depressed they were.

Occasionally, reports appear of persistent, severe memory loss after ECT (Donahue, 2000). Such reports are often sensationalized by the media and anti-psychiatry groups. Adverse cognitive outcomes are much less likely in the modern age, with contemporary ECT techniques, than they were in the distant past.

Headache, Muscle Aches, and Nausea

Headache

A substantial proportion of patients report headache following ECT. This side effect may be related to the contraction of the temporalis and masseter muscles or to the cerebral hemodynamic changes that accompany the treatment. Although the exact etiology of the headache is unclear, it is typically transient and responds well to acetaminophen, aspirin, or other nonsteroidal anti-inflammatory agents. Rarely, triptans or opiates may be required (Markowitz et al., 2001).

A common treatment strategy is the administration of 30 mg intravenous ketorolac (Toradol) just before the ECT procedure. Generally, this is not done at the first treatment; rather, if the patient reports a significant headache after the first treatment, ketorolac may be offered before subsequent treatments. Another preemptive analgesia strategy is to give, for example, 600 mg ibuprofen (Motrin) po 2 hours before ECT.

Muscle Aches

Diffuse myalgias are most commonly seen after the first ECT session and then subside following subsequent treatments. This symptom is likely due to muscle fasciculations from succinylcholine. Typically, the myalgias are transient and respond well to the same symptomatic treatment used for headaches. If myalgias persist after subsequent treatments and the patient's muscular block is adequate, the practitioner should consider lowering the succinylcholine dose or, in rare situations, blocking fasciculations by pretreatment with a small dose of a nondepolarizing muscle relaxant.

Nausea

A minority of patients are nauseated after ECT. This side effect may be related to the anesthetic, the seizure itself, or air in the stomach from assisted ventilation. When it is a regular occurrence, nausea may be treated with intravenous ondansetron (Zofran) 4 mg, given shortly before the procedure. Ondansetron may also be given IV or po after the treatment for persistent nausea. Drinking a carbonated beverage, such as, ginger ale, is also often helpful.

References

Abrams, R. 2002. *Electroconvulsive Therapy*. New York: Oxford University Press.

Donahue, A. B. 2000. Electroconvulsive therapy and memory loss: a personal journey. *J ECT*, **16**, 133–43.

Loo, C. 2008. Cognitive outcomes in electroconvulsive therapy: optimizing current clinical practice and researching future strategies. *J ECT*, **24**, 1–2.

Markowitz, J. S., Kellner, C. H., Devane, C. L., et al. 2001. Intranasal sumatriptan in post-ECT headache: results of an open-label trial. *J ECT*, **17**, 280–3.

Semkovska, M., & McLoughlin, D. M. 2010. Objective cognitive performance associated with electroconvulsive therapy for depression: a systematic review and meta-analysis. *Biol Psychiatry*, **68**, 568–77.

Squire, L. R. 1986. Memory functions as affected by electroconvulsive therapy. *Ann N Y Acad Sci*, **462**, 307–14.

Electroconvulsive Therapy (ECT): The ECT Service

Staffing and Administration

The electroconvulsive therapy (ECT) staff consists of a multidisciplinary team working together to provide optimal patient care. The ECT-trained psychiatrist leads the team, working in a collaborative relationship with anesthesia and nursing personnel.

Perhaps the most important issue in ECT-related patient care is the quality of the working relationship between psychiatrist and anesthetist. The development of a mutually respectful, trusting relationship is as important as a good intravenous line! Such a relationship takes some time to develop and is facilitated by having only a few anesthesia personnel rotate through the treatment suite and by reaching agreement regarding consistency of the anesthetic plan among all staff members.

Nursing staff play a key role in the delivery of ECT. Depending on how a particular ECT service is staffed and organized, nursing roles may include both administrative and direct clinical care responsibilities. One designated nurse should be in charge of all nursing issues related to ECT. She or he should supervise the other recovery or treatment area nurse(s) and see to it that the specific nursing functions of the treatment procedure are carried out. These include performing the "time out" patient and procedure recognition process (where mandated), recording of vital signs and medications given, and insertion of the bite block. Other nursing functions may include other medical record keeping, patient education, and clinical assessment, as well as responsibility for maintaining equipment and supplies in the treatment room.

As the leader of the treatment team, the psychiatrist is responsible for maintaining the medical standards and professional atmosphere of the ECT suite. To this end, he or she should feel comfortable in politely reminding his or her colleagues that voices should be kept low and that there is no place for discussion of other "interesting cases" within earshot of patients. At all times,

Brain Stimulation in Psychiatry: ECT, DBS, TMS, and Other Modalities, Charles H. Kellner. Published by Cambridge University Press. © Charles H. Kellner, 2012.

the overriding principle should be that patients will be treated in the way we would want to be treated were we in their situation.

The ECT Suite

Ideally, ECT should be done in a suite of rooms specially designed to provide separate treatment, recovery, and waiting areas. Adequate space should be available to provide privacy for patients and a calm, quiet environment for post-treatment recovery. Waiting areas for family members should be nearby and hospitable. The experience of having ECT should be similar to a visit to a well-run private internist's or dentist's office.

The location of the ECT suite is also very important. There is no absolute need to do ECT in an expensive operating room or general post-anesthesia recovery area. Such areas tend to be busy, hectic, public, and potentially frightening to patients. A location on the psychiatry unit or a separate area in an outpatient surgery facility is preferable. In some instances, consideration should be given to treating a severely medically ill patient in the hospital operating room or main recovery room suite, for optimum access to emergency equipment and medical staff.

The equipment necessary for an ECT suite, well described in the report of the American Psychiatric Association (APA) Task Force on ECT (American Psychiatric Association, 2001) includes the following:

- Suction and oxygen are needed in both treatment and recovery areas. An anesthesia device, although preferred by many, is not necessary, and wall oxygen with disposable breathing circuits and masks is fully satisfactory.
- Pulse oximeters should be available for both treatment and recovery areas.
- An ECG/automatic blood pressure monitor should be located in the treatment room.
- A nerve stimulator should be available.
- A fully stocked drug and emergency equipment cabinet should be at hand in the treatment room, and responsibility for deciding on which drugs to include should be shared by the psychiatric and anesthesia staff. Restocking of supplies is usually the responsibility of the nursing staff.
- Finally, the ECT device, with all necessary supplies (including a copy of the instruction manual for quick reference) should be located on a countertop or a cart near the treatment stretcher.

Record Keeping

Documentation of the ECT evaluation and treatment process is essential for good patient care and for medicolegal purposes. The two primary records to be kept are the patient's medical record and the ECT service's record.

The Medical Record

The patient's medical record should contain the ECT consultation sheet, detailing the indications for treatment, pertinent medical issues, and recommendations about consent. All the required pre-ECT workup should be in the medical record, as well as the completed consent form. There should be a procedure note for each ECT treatment. This note should include doses of treatment medications, electrode placement, treatment number, stimulus parameters and dose, motor and EEG seizure durations, and any complications noted and their management. The anesthesia staff and the recovery nursing staff should also include appropriate documentation of the patient's clinical status during treatment and recovery, including serial vital signs. The ECT team's appraisal of the patient's clinical status and the plan for ongoing management should be included in the chart at least once a week during the ECT course.

The ECT Service's Record

The ECT service may maintain a separate record of the pre-ECT evaluation, procedure parameters, clinical response and/or complications, and recommendations for continuation therapy. Such separate ECT records facilitate retrieval of ECT information that may be needed for future patient care, for transmittal to other hospital facilities, or for monitoring trends in ECT practice. As the recording of medical records becomes increasingly electronic, it is likely that both clinical and research ECT databases will be fully computerized in the near future.

Reference

American Psychiatric Association. 2001. *Task Force on Electroconvulsive Therapy. The Practice of Electroconvulsive Therapy: Recommendations for Treatment, Training, and Privileging.* Washington, DC: American Psychiatric Association.

Electroconvulsive Therapy (ECT): Special Issues

Stigma

Stigma remains the biggest impediment to the acceptance of ECT. The burden of the abuses of the past, irrational fears of the electrical stimulus, and exaggerated concerns about memory loss all contribute to the stigma surrounding ECT. An example of how destructive this stigma can be is the despicable discrediting of 1972 vice-presidential candidate Thomas Eagleton when his history of ECT treatment was revealed. Fortunately, courageous efforts to counter stigma also exist; one example is television personality Dick Cavett's disclosure that ECT effectively reversed his serious depression. In recent years, many patients have spoken and written courageously about their positive experiences with ECT (Manning, 1994; Hersh, 2011).

Perhaps the best way to counter the stigma surrounding ECT is to educate ourselves well and to insist on high standards in the performance of ECT. We hope that this book is helpful in achieving those goals.

Malpractice Litigation and Insurance

Because of the safety of the procedure, ECT generates remarkably little in the way of malpractice litigation. This topic has been very well covered by Richard Abrams in his textbook (Abrams, 2002). He provides a list of commonsense rules of good medical practice that will help reduce the (already low) risk of malpractice litigation.

In recent years, there have been several instances of the elimination of insurance surcharges for ECT because of the absence of successful suits. When these surcharges were challenged, it was demonstrated that, in fact, ECT did not contribute to higher malpractice insurance costs.

Research

The extensive ECT literature attests to a 70-year history of productive clinical and basic science research in ECT. We know a tremendous amount about many

Brain Stimulation in Psychiatry: ECT, DBS, TMS, and Other Modalities, Charles H. Kellner. Published by Cambridge University Press. © Charles H. Kellner, 2012.

aspects of ECT (Fink, 2011; Sienaert, 2011; Loo et al., 2006). However, we need to know much more, both about the way ECT works and about how to reduce its side effects.

Important areas of ongoing research include the following:

- Mechanism(s) of action
- Prediction of responders to right unilateral vs. bilateral electrode placement
- Adjunctive drugs to reduce cognitive effects
- Determination of optimal stimulus parameters
- Safety of ECT-drug combinations
- Continuation/maintenance ECT and medication treatments after ECT
- Neuropsychiatric indications for ECT, including Parkinson's disease

References

Abrams, R. 2002. *Electroconvulsive Therapy*. Oxford, New York: Oxford University Press.

Fink, M. 2011. Electroconvulsive therapy resurrected: its successes and promises after 75 years. *Canad J Psychiatry. Revue canadienne de psychiatrie*, **56**, 3–4.

Hersh, J. 2011. *Struck by Living: From Depression to Hope*. Austin, TX, Greenleaf Book Group Press.

Loo, C. K., Schweitzer, I., & Pratt, C. 2006. Recent advances in optimizing electroconvulsive therapy. *The Australian and New Zealand J Psychiatry*, **40**, 632–8.

Manning, M. 1994. *Undercurrents : A Therapist's Reckoning With Her Own Depression*. New York: HarperCollins Pub.

Sienaert, P. 2011. What we have learned about electroconvulsive therapy and its relevance for the practising psychiatrist. *Canadian J Psychiatry. Revue Canadienne de Psychiatrie*, **56**, 5–12.

Chapter 9

Deep Brain Stimulation (DBS)

Wayne K. Goodman, MD and Ron L. Alterman, MD

Portions of this chapter were adapted with permission from Goodman (2012)

Basic Concepts

Deep brain stimulation (DBS) is a novel approach to electrical stimulation of the brain that has revolutionized the treatment of medically refractory movement disorders including essential tremor (ET), Parkinson's disease (PD), and torsion dystonia (Table 9.1). The successful treatment of these disorders has generated excitement about the possibility of using DBS to treat refractory psychiatric ailments such as obsessive-compulsive disorder (OCD), Tourette syndrome, and major depressive disorder (MDD). Presently in the United States, the treatment of OCD with DBS is approved under a Humanitarian Device Exemption (HDE); all other uses for psychiatric disorders are currently considered to be "off-label." At the time that this manuscript was prepared, Medtronic Inc. (Minneapolis, MN) was the only manufacturer with FDA approval to sell a DBS system in the United States. St. Jude Neurological, Inc. (Plano, TX), has received approval to market its DBS system for the treatment of PD and ET in Europe; FDA approval for these applications is pending.

DBS involves the surgical implantation of one or more "leads" into the substance of the brain by means of burr holes that are made in the region of the coronal suture. These leads (thin flexible cables equipped with a series of electrode contacts at the end) are then connected to extension cables, which are tunneled under the skin from the cranium to the anterior chest wall where they are connected to a programmable pulse generator (PG), which produces the therapeutic electrical current (see Figures 9.1 and 9.2). Therapeutic success depends upon identifying the proper brain target for stimulation, accurately targeting that site with the lead, and delivering an electrical current of appropriate amplitude, pattern, duration, and frequency to modulate neural activity in an efficacious manner.

The goal of this chapter is to familiarize the reader with DBS technology, the implantation surgery, a general approach to programming the device, and the preliminary clinical results treating psychiatric illness. Unlike ECT, DBS for

Brain Stimulation in Psychiatry: ECT, DBS, TMS, and Other Modalities, Charles H. Kellner. Published by Cambridge University Press. © Charles H. Kellner, 2012.

Table 9.1. Status of Deep Brain Stimulation

Description of Procedure	Uses: Established or Investigational	FDA Regulatory Status	Safety/Tolerability of Procedure
Lead(s) implanted in brain anatomic target through burr hole(s) in cranium and locked in place	Movement Disorders Psychiatric Disorders: • OCD	Approved for Essential Tremor Approved for refractory Parkinson's Disease	Invasive: requires craniotomy and implantation of electrodes directly in brain parenchyma
Extension wires tunneled under skin and connected to pulse generator(s) implanted under skin of chest	• Depression • Tourette Syndrome	Limited approval under HDE for: • Dystonia	Risk of serious adverse events including intracerebral hemorrhage (~2%) and infection (~10%)
Programming of device settings performed wirelessly		• Intractable OCD	Over 75,000 operations performed worldwide for movement disorders

Abbreviations: OCD=Obsessive-Compulsive Disorder; FDA=Food & Drug Administration; HDE=Human Device Exemption.

psychiatric disorders is in its infancy; but it is hoped that on going pivotal trials will test its efficacy and safety in the near future.

Pre-operative Evaluation

DBS is best administered by a multidisciplinary team consisting of a neuro-surgeon with expertise in stereotactic surgery, one or more psychiatrists who are responsible for programming the device(s) once it is implanted, a neuro-psychologist, and additional ancillary staff (e.g., nurse practitioners) as required. As the expert in the treatment of psychiatric disorders, the psychia-trist should take the lead role in this collaboration, determining the candidacy for surgical intervention, and managing the patient's care once the devices are implanted. The surgeon's role is to ensure that there are no medical contra-indications to surgery, perform the operation deftly, and manage any surgical complications that may arise.

Presently, DBS should only be considered for patients with severe OCD, TS, or MDD whose symptoms are inadequately controlled with standard therapies for that disorder including medications and Cognitive Behavioral Therapy (CBT) in the case of OCD. Medication trials should be of sufficient dose and duration to ensure that the medication is truly ineffective or cannot be toler-ated. Once it is determined that the patient is truly disabled and refractory to standard treatment, referral can be made for surgery. The surgeon must ensure that the patient is medically able to undergo the procedure. In addition, select patients may require detailed neurocognitive assessment to rule out early dementia, which can be exacerbated by the procedure. Finally, the patient must be competent to participate in the informed consent process and must be made to understand the long-term commitment that is required for this therapy to be successful.

The DBS Device

A DBS device consists of four components:

1. One or more **stimulating leads**, which are implanted stereotactically within the desired brain target(s) and are equipped with one or more electrodes or "contacts" through which electrical current is delivered to the target. These wires are thin and flexible, allowing them to move with the brain for safe chronic implantation. Presently, leads are comprised of four cylindrical contacts with varied spacing; however, future systems may have more electrode contacts and the contacts will be segmented, allowing for greater control shaping the therapeutic field.
2. A **locking device**, which is secured to the skull and both anchors the lead and covers the burr hole through which the lead is placed.
3. A programmable **pulse generator** (PG), which is placed under the skin of the chest wall or abdomen like a cardiac pacemaker and delivers the therapeutic current. These may be "single channel" devices where one stimulator serves one lead or "dual channel" devices, where one stimulator serves two leads. These devices may come equipped with standard batteries or may be rechargeable. Rechargeable devices are smaller and will last longer; however, they are more expensive and the patient must remember to recharge the device regularly or risk having it turn off with loss of therapeutic effect.
4. One or two **extension cables**, heftier than the leads, which are tunneled under the skin and connect the PG to the implanted brain lead(s).

The Surgical Procedure

DBS devices are implanted in two stages. During the first stage, the lead wire(s) is implanted within the desired target(s). This may be accomplished with a variety of "stereotactic" techniques, which allow surgeons to place probes deep within the brain by means of small cranial openings. These techniques use computerized image guidance (CT and/or MRI) with or without intra-operative physiological refinement. Traditionally, a stereotactic headframe is used to accomplish this task. Newer mini-frame techniques are gaining popularity; however, they do not yet have the long-term track record of stereotactic frames. In most cases implantation of the lead(s) is performed with the patient awake so that the surgical team can monitor the patient's responses to stimulation in the operating room. This is possible, of course, because the brain is insensate to pain and so local anesthetic applied to the scalp makes this procedure no more painful (albeit more stressful and higher risk) than a trip to the endodontist. A brief description of the lead implantation procedure follows.

Stage 1: Implantation of the Brain Leads

After administering a local anesthetic, the stereotactic headframe is applied rigidly to the patient's skull using MRI-compatible pins. Rigid fixation of the frame to the cranium is critical as any movement of the frame relative to the patient's brain will result in a misplaced lead at best and a serious neurological injury or death at worst. After applying the frame, a "localizer box" is placed on the frame around the patient's head. This box contains columns of copper sulfate solution, which leave visible fiducial marks on the targeting MRI or CT scan. These marks define stereotactic space and allow for the creation of a Cartesian coordinate system from which the three-dimensional coordinates for a given target can be determined. Both because the frame is applied somewhat differently each time it is used and because the human brain is highly variable in shape and size, the coordinates for a given anatomical structure will vary each time the device is used. The targeting images are uploaded onto a computer workstation in the operating room for surgical planning. The targeting software is used to determine the coordinates for the desired target as well as the safest trajectory to the target.

The patient is positioned supine with the head elevated ~30°, much like a reclining chair. The frame is fixed to the table immobilizing the patient's head both for safety and the surgeon's ease. Following a standard prep and drape the desired target coordinates and angles of approach are set on the frame and the operation begins. A small incision is made in the frontal scalp, centered on the desired trajectory. This incision rests behind the hairline for most patients and is therefore not visible once the hair grows back. A burr hole is then drilled in the frontal bone, again centered on the planned trajectory. The anchoring device is then secured to the skull. The dura is opened exposing the cortex, a small area of which is gently coagulated and incised to facilitate insertion of the blunt-tipped guide tube. This thin guide tube (outer diameter ~1.8 mm) is then inserted along the desired trajectory to a point ~10 mm shy of the desired target. For some deep brain targets (particularly deep nuclei), the surgeon may elect to perform single-cell microelectrode recording to confirm proper targeting; however, this technique is not as useful for identifying the predominantly white matter structures that are currently being targeted to treat psychiatric disorders.

The DBS lead is then inserted through the guide tube to the target. The extracranial end of the lead wire is connected to a temporary extension, the other end of which is connected to an external stimulator so that test stimulation may be performed. During test stimulation, the examining physician (operating surgeon and/or psychiatrist) examines the patient while administering stimulation by means of each of the contacts on the implanted lead. Unlike tremor, symptoms of OCD and MDD may not respond to stimulation for weeks or months and so an immediate beneficial response is not expected. One possible exception is the smile reflex, which was first described by Okun et al. (2004). They noted that some patients undergoing stimulation at the Anterior Limb of the Internal Capsule (ALIC) spontaneously smile during test stimulation. They propose that this may be a positive outcome predictor for OCD; but to date, this hypothesis remains unproven.

Following test stimulation, the lead is anchored in place with the locking mechanism that was attached to the skull earlier in the procedure. Intra-operative fluoroscopy is used to demonstrate electrode position relative to the frame during this process so that the surgeon does not inadvertently displace the lead. The locking device is then capped, covering the burr hole site. The remaining length of lead wire is left in the sub-galeal space and the incision is sutured closed.

After both leads are implanted the patient is brought back to Radiology where a CT or MRI scan is performed. This post-operative scan documents the anatomical position of the implanted leads and demonstrates whether or not an intracerebral hemorrhage has occurred during the procedure. If the electrodes are well-positioned, there has been no hemorrhage, and the patient is well neurologically, the patient may be returned to the operating room for stage 2: implantation of the extension cables and pulse generator(s). This second stage procedure may be delayed; however, patients cannot benefit from the implanted leads until the remainder of the system is implanted and activated.

Stage 2: Implantation of the Extension Cables and Pulse Generator(s)

The second stage is performed under general anesthesia. During this procedure a sub-cutaneous pocket is made either in the infraclavicular region or, less often, in the abdomen. The free end of the lead wires are accessed in the sub-galeal space, the extension cable(s) are tunneled underneath the skin from the chest (or abdominal) incision to the cranial incision and the components are connected, completing the circuit. The surgeon must ensure that all of the connections are clean and dry so there will be neither short nor open circuits. The incisions are sutured closed and the patient is monitored overnight on the Neurosurgery Ward or ICU as dictated clinically.

Activation and Programming of the DBS Devices

Device programming typically begins one or two weeks following surgery, allowing time for the surgical wounds to heal and for the patient to return to his/her baseline state. The pulse generator is programmed telemetrically using a hand held device. The treating physician determines the following stimulation parameters: (1) signal intensity; (2) the active electrode contact(s); (3) whether unipolar (i.e., the stimulator serves as the anode and one or more lead contacts serve as the active cathode) or bipolar (i.e., both the cathode and anode are contacts on the lead) will be used; (4) the stimulation frequency; and (5) the pulse width. As the number of different possible permutations is enormous, programming algorithms built on prior clinical experience are followed to render this task more manageable. Moreover, the significant delay between the onset of stimulation and clinical response makes programming more challenging. For these reasons, optimizing DBS settings for psychiatric disorders is currently more art than science and requires a great deal of patience on the part of both the patient and programmer.

The patient is given a similar hand held device with limited functionality to take home. The PG(s) can be inactivated inadvertently by strong magnetic fields in the modern environment (e.g., metal detectors, refrigerator magnets). The programmer given to the patients can check and restore operation of the PG should it be inactivated. Conversely, if adverse stimulation effects occur, or if the patient needs to undergo a diagnostic test such as EKG, the patient can turn off the PG. As a safeguard, the patient cannot change other parameters that alter the stimulation field or intensity. For example, it would be problematic if the patient could self-induce hypomania.

To date, studies of DBS in neuropsychiatric disorders have used continuous stimulation settings though for some paroxysmal psychiatric disorders (e.g., TS and OCD), "on demand" or even cycled stimulation might be more desirable. Closed-loop devices are under development in which output to the target is responsive to input from the same or another brain region.

If DBS treatment is unsuccessful, the hardware can be explanted. The available data from post-mortem examination of brains from patients with implanted electrodes suggest that the pathological changes produced by chronic DBS are limited to minimal gliosis along the electrode track (DiLorenzo et al., 2010).

DBS in Obsessive-Compulsive Disorder (OCD)

DBS at the ALIC was first reported to be a promising intervention for OCD in a 1999 publication by Nuttin et al. (1999). The roots of DBS stimulation for OCD can be traced to positive experiences with both gamma capsulotomy and thermolytic ablative surgery in this brain region (Mindus et al., 1999). The

Gamma Knife studies at Brown University suggested that lesions in the most ventral region of the ALIC, extending inferiorly into the ventral striatum, improved outcome (Goodman and Insel, 2009). DBS was proposed as a reversible alternative to ablation as it was generally believed that high-frequency electrical stimulation (on the order of 130 Hz) would produce "functional ablation" of the same target. It was expected that high-frequency DBS would interrupt the pathways that mediated OCD behaviors. Functional brain imaging studies in patients with OCD provided an independent rationale for DBS therapy in the region of the ventral ALIC (Greenberg et al., 2008). Pathways coursing through the ALIC have been implicated in neurocircuitry models of OCD (Greenberg et al., 2010b).

Following the initial report of Nuttin et al. (1999), several other groups have reported on their experience in intractable OCD with DBS of the ALIC (Abelson et al., 2005) or neighboring brain regions, including the ventral capsule/ventral striatum (VC/VS) (Goodman et al., 2010; Greenberg et al., 2010a) and nucleus accumbens (NAc) (Denys et al., 2010; Huff et al., 2010). Many of the findings are from uncontrolled, open-label studies or case reports. Several studies included a double-blind period with an on-off phase (Abelson et al., 2005; Denys et al., 2010) or staggered-onset design (Goodman et al., 2010). The two most rigorous studies used a double-blind sham-controlled design with 3-month treatment arms (Huff et al., 2010; Mallet et al., 2008). The largest long-term open-label follow-up study included 26 patients that were followed for a mean of 31.4 months. Using stringent criteria, >60% of these patients showed a response (Greenberg et al., 2010a). A review by de Koning et al., concluded that the overall response rate was over 50% across all published papers on the various DBS targets (de Koning et al., 2011). Lower response rates were seen with subthalamic nucleus (STN) stimulation (Mallet et al., 2008) and unilateral stimulation to the NAc (Huff et al., 2010).

DBS in Depression

Mayberg's research group published open-label outcome data on 20 patients with treatment-resistant depression (TRD) who underwent DBS to the subcallosal cingulate gyrus (SCG) (Kennedy et al., 2011). During extended follow-up (3–6 years), the response rate was 55% for the last available study visit in the intent-to-treat sample (Kennedy et al., 2011). Three patients were explanted at their request due to lack of efficacy. The high rate of mortality associated with TRD is underscored by the death of two patients by suicide. Neither of these deaths was attributed to device malfunction or effects of stimulation (Kennedy et al., 2011).

Malone et al. (2009) reported outcome and safety data from an open-label multicenter study of VC/VS stimulation in 15 patients with chronic, severe TRD. The criteria for treatment-resistance were stringent and included failure to respond to an adequate trial of electroconvulsive therapy. After 6 months of continuous stimulation, 40% of the patients were classified as responders. The procedures were generally well tolerated.

Adverse Effects

Potential complications of DBS can be categorized as related to (1) surgical implantation, (2) device failure, and (3) stimulation. The first two categories are well known due to the more than 75,000 DBS implants that have been performed worldwide, mostly to treat movement disorders. In contrast, adverse effects induced by stimulation (or its interruption) at the targets used to treat psychiatric disorders are just being described.

Complications of Surgery

The most daunting risk of DBS therapy is that of stroke and/or hemorrhage during implantation of the DBS leads. Hemorrhage rates of 0–10% are reported in the literature (Bronstein et al., 2011), though larger series report rates of ~2% (Foltynie and Hariz, 2010; Follett et al., 2010). Depending on the size and location, these hemorrhages may be inconsequential or may cause a variety of neurological deficits or death. The risk of hemorrhage may be correlated to larger numbers of microelectrode recording trajectories (used to electrophysiologically identify the therapeutic target) (Foltynie and Hariz, 2010; Mikos et al., 2010) and implantation trajectories that traverse the sulci and/or the lateral ventricles (Gologorsky et al., 2011; Sansur et al., 2007). We would expect a very low risk of hemorrhage (1–2% or less) in DBS procedures for psychiatric disorders because the ventricles are easy to avoid when approaching these targets, and target localization is not dependent on microelectrode recording. Nevertheless, so long as the brain parenchyma is penetrated, hemorrhage and its potentially disastrous sequelae will remain a risk of these procedures.

The second most feared complication of DBS surgery is post-operative confusion. The risk of confusion is increased in elderly patients (Doshi, 2011), particularly those with PD (of which dementia may be a component) and in patients undergoing bilateral contemporaneous implants. We expect that this also will be a rare complication in patients with refractory OCD and MDD who will be younger, on average, than PD patients, and who are not suffering from disorders of which dementia is a feature.

The most common complication of DBS surgery is infection, which is reported to occur in 0–15% of cases (Bronstein et al., 2011). In theory, spread of an infection along the implanted brain lead could result in meningitis, cerebritis, or brain abscess; but in reality, these are rare occurrences. In our experience, most infections occur at the chest pocket, allowing for preservation of the brain lead if one acts quickly to remove the infected PG and extension.

Complications Related to Chronic Hardware Implantation

The Medtronic Activa™ deep brain stimulation system has been commercially available in the U.S. and E.U. for almost 15 years, so the long-term risks associated with implanting these devices are quite evident. Overall, chronic implantation of these devices is well tolerated. Although hardware-related complications are reported to occur in as many as 25% of patients at some point in time, the annualized risk is approximately 4% and most of the complications are not life-threatening and readily managed (Doshi, 2011; Boviatsis et al., 2010; Paluzzi et al., 2006; Oh et al., 2002). In our experience and that reported by others, erosion of the scalp tissue overlying the burr hole cap is the most significant long-term complication of the implanted device and is most commonly observed in balding men and the elderly, whose scalps are more atrophic.

These devices are battery powered and must, therefore, be replaced periodically. The effective life of a device depends on the amount of current that is required to achieve optimal clinical effect. This effective life may be as long as 7 or 8 years in patients with Essential Tremor who turn their devices off at night, or as short as 12 months in some patients receiving VC/VS stimulation, where very high amplitudes and constant stimulation may be required. And while battery replacement surgery is a short, simple ambulatory procedure during which only the PG pocket is accessed, it is an expensive surgery and frequent battery change surgeries pose both health and financial burdens. The advent of PGs with rechargeable batteries will remedy this problem while introducing a new burden: the time spent recharging the devices. Hopefully, advances in our understanding of how DBS works may lead to improved stimulation paradigms that both improve clinical outcomes and decrease electrical energy requirements. In 4 patients who were implanted under the HDE for OCD, we have been able to conserve battery life by having the patients turn off their PGs during sleep (Goodman and Alterman, 2011).

Conclusions

The therapeutic effects of DBS have been reported in approximately 100 cases of OCD (de Koning et al., 2011) and 50 cases of TRD for seven (five common) anatomic targets (Greenberg et al., 2010a). Although these published reports differ with respect to study design, sample size, subject characteristics, and outcome measurement, the overall response rate appears to exceed 50% in OCD for DBS targets in the area of the ventral striatum and nucleus accumbens (de Koning et al., 2011). In TRD, more than 50% of patients responded during acute and long-term (range = 3–6 years) bilateral electrical stimulation of the SCG (n = 20) (Kennedy et al., 2011). The response rate of TRD to VC/VS stimulation appears lower (Malone et al., 2009). Despite the drawbacks of open-label follow-up data, the maintenance of response several years after implantation is encouraging for several DBS targets in OCD (de Koning et al., 2011) and SCG stimulation in MDD (Kennedy et al., 2011).

The extant literature on DBS for psychiatric disorders reports a low rate of serious adverse events related to surgery or hardware malfunction. An exception was an intracerebral brain hemorrhage that produced a permanent finger palsy in one patient undergoing STN DBS for OCD (Mallet et al., 2008). Ongoing brain stimulation was generally well tolerated across multiple targets for both OCD and TRD. Some unique, target- and stimulation-specific adverse effects were observed, such as, hypomania. Stimulation of the VC/VS-NAc region has been associated with acute induction of elevated mood and affect that ranges from a smile to laughter to hypomania depending on the stimulation parameters (Okun et al., 2004; Goodman et al., 2010; Greenberg et al., 2010b; Chang et al., 2010). Unpleasant adverse behavioral effects such as panic attacks have also been observed with DBS in the VC/VS-NAc region at the most ventral contacts (Shapira et al., 2006). In all reported cases, undesirable effects of DBS on mood, including hypomania, were reversible with changes in device settings. Apart from mild forgetfulness (de Koning et al., 2011) reported in some cases, DBS has not been associated with clinically significant changes in cognitive function during treatment of either OCD (Dougherty et al., 2002) or MDD (McNeely et al., 2008). Accidental device cessation or battery depletion can result in depressed mood or worsening of OCD (Greenberg et al., 2010b). Two completed suicides in one study of TRD were attributed to the underlying disorder, not DBS device failure (Kennedy et al., 2011).

Limitations of the published data on DBS in OCD and MDD include the small sample sizes (many are single case reports) and open-label design of most studies. Only a few studies, all of them in OCD, used a blinded on-off phase and only two included a blinded treatment arm as long as 3 months (Goodman and Alterman, 2012). Randomized sham-controlled studies with sufficiently long blinded phases (preferably at least 6 months) are warranted in both OCD and MDD. Specifically, further research is needed to (1) test the efficacy and safety of DBS, (2) compare targets, (3) optimize device settings, and (4) identify predictors of response so that the most appropriate patients can be selected. Equally important is achieving a better understanding of the mechanisms of action of DBS in psychiatric disorders so that less invasive interventions can be developed.

Given the checkered history of "psychosurgery" and the fact that DBS is an invasive and a high-risk procedure, the public needs reassurance that "the clinical use of DBS in [psychiatric disorders] will not overstep the bounds of empirical evidence" (Goodman and Insel, 2009). Questions have already been raised about whether the FDA should have approved an HDE for DBS in OCD (Fins et al., 2011). Indeed, the efficacy of VC/VS DBS for intractable OCD has not been established. Unfortunately, adequately powered randomized clinical

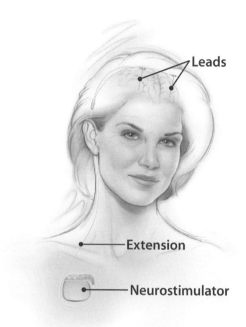

Figure 9.1. A DBS system in place. Image courtesy of Medtronic.

Leads

Extension

Neurostimulator

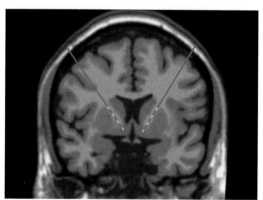

Figure 9.2. Coronal image showing projected placement of leads in a patient undergoing DBS of the anterior limb of the internal capsule for major depressive disorder. Image courtesy of Medtronic.

trials of DBS in OCD may not be feasible (e.g., difficulty recruiting subjects and high cost to sponsor for a limited market). In contrast, studies of DBS for TRD are currently underway that should be large enough to answer questions about both efficacy and safety of this intervention for specific anatomic targets.

References

Abelson, J. L., Curtis, G. C., Sagher, O., et al. 2005. Deep brain stimulation for refractory obsessive-compulsive disorder. *Biol Psychiatry*, **57**, 510–6.

Boviatsis, E. J., Stavrinou, L. C., Themistocleous, M., Kouyialis, A. T., & Sakas, D. E. 2010. Surgical and hardware complications of deep brain stimulation. A seven-year experience and review of the literature. *Acta Neurochir (Wien)*, **152**, 2053–62.

Bronstein, J. M., Tagliati, M., Alterman, R. L., et al. 2011. Deep brain stimulation for Parkinson disease: an expert consensus and review of key issues. *Arch Neurol*, **68**, 165.

Chang, C. H., Chen, S. Y., Hsiao, Y. L., Tsai, S. T., & Tsai, H. C. 2010. Hypomania with hypersexuality following bilateral anterior limb stimulation in obsessive-compulsive disorder. *J Neurosurg*, **112**, 1299–300.

de Koning, P. P., Figee, M., van den Munckhof, P., Schuurman, P. R., & Denys, D. 2011. Current status of deep brain stimulation for obsessive-compulsive disorder: a clinical review of different targets. *Curr Psychiatry Rep*, **13**, 274–82.

Denys, D., Mantione, M., Figee, M., et al. 2010. Deep brain stimulation of the nucleus accumbens for treatment-refractory obsessive-compulsive disorder. *Arch Gen Psychiatry*, **67**, 1061–8.

DiLorenzo, D. J., Jankovic, J., Simpson, R. K., Takei, H., & Powell, S. Z. 2010. Long-term deep brain stimulation for essential tremor: 12-year clinicopathologic follow-up. *Mov Disord*, **25**, 232–8.

Doshi, P. K. 2011. Long-term surgical and hardware-related complications of deep brain stimulation. *Stereotact Funct Neurosurg*, **89**, 89–95.

Dougherty, D. D., Baer, L., Cosgrove, G. R., et al. 2002. Prospective long-term follow-up of 44 patients who received cingulotomy for treatment-refractory obsessive-compulsive disorder. *Am J Psychiatry*, **159**, 269–75.

Fins, J. J., Mayberg, H. S., Nuttin, B., et al. 2011. Misuse of the FDA's humanitarian device exemption in deep brain stimulation for obsessive-compulsive disorder. *Health Aff (Millwood)*. **30**, 302–11.

Follett, K. A., Weaver, F. M., Stern, M., et al. 2010. Pallidal versus subthalamic deep-brain stimulation for Parkinson's disease. *N Engl J Med*, **362**, 2077–91.

Foltynie, T., & Hariz, M. I. 2010. Surgical management of Parkinson's disease. *Expert Rev Neurother*, **10**, 903–14.

Gologorsky, Y., Ben-Haim, S., Moshier, E. L., et al. 2011. Transgressing the ventricular wall during subthalamic deep brain stimulation surgery for Parkinson disease increases the risk of adverse neurological sequelae. *Neurosurgery*, **69**, 294–9; discussion 9–300.

Goodman, W. G., & Alterman, R. Inactivation of deep brain stimulation during sleep in four patients with obsessive-compulsive disorder. unpublished data. 2011.

Goodman, W. K., & Alterman R. L. 2012. Deep brain stimulation for intractable psychiatric disorders. *Annu Rev Med*, **63**, 1–14.

Goodman, W. K., Foote, K. D., Greenberg, B. D., et al. 2010. Deep brain stimulation for intractable obsessive compulsive disorder: pilot study using a blinded, staggered-onset design. *Biol Psychiatry*, **67**, 535–42.

Goodman, W. K., & Insel, T. R. 2009. Deep brain stimulation in psychiatry: concentrating on the road ahead. *Biol Psychiatry*, **65**, 263–6.

Greenberg, B. D., Askland, K. D., & Carpenter, L. L. 2008. The evolution of deep brain stimulation for neuropsychiatric disorders. *Front Biosci*, **13**, 4638–48.

Greenberg, B. D., Gabriels, L. A., Malone, D. A., Jr., et al. 2010a. Deep brain stimulation of the ventral internal capsule/ventral striatum for obsessive-compulsive disorder: worldwide experience. *Mol Psychiatry*, **15**, 64–79.

Greenberg, B. D., Rauch, S. L., & Haber, S. N. 2010b. Invasive circuitry-based neurotherapeutics: stereotactic ablation and deep brain stimulation for OCD. *Neuropsychopharmacology*, **35**, 317–36.

Huff, W., Lenartz, D., Schormann, M., et al. 2010. Unilateral deep brain stimulation of the nucleus accumbens in patients with treatment-resistant obsessive-compulsive disorder: outcomes after one year. *Clin Neurol Neurosurg*, **112**, 137–43.

Kennedy, S. H., Giacobbe, P., Rizvi, S. J., et al. 2011. Deep brain stimulation for treatment-resistant depression: follow-up after 3 to 6 years. *Am J Psychiatry*, **168**, 502–10.

Mallet, L., Polosan, M., Jaafari, N., et al. 2008. Subthalamic nucleus stimulation in severe obsessive-compulsive disorder. *N Engl J Med*. **359**, 2121–34.

Malone, D. A., Jr., Dougherty, D. D., Rezai, A. R., et al. 2009. Deep brain stimulation of the ventral capsule/ventral striatum for treatment-resistant depression. *Biol Psychiatry*, **65**, 267–75.

McNeely, H. E., Mayberg, H. S., Lozano, A. M., & Kennedy, S. H. 2008. Neuropsychological impact of Cg25 deep brain stimulation for treatment-resistant depression: preliminary results over 12 months. *J Nerv Ment Dis*. **196**, 405–10.

Mikos, A., Pavon, J., Bowers, D., et al. 2010. Factors related to extended hospital stays following deep brain stimulation for Parkinson's disease. *Parkinsonism Relat Disord*, **16**, 324–8.

Mindus, P., Edman, G., & Andréewitch, S. 1999. A prospective, long-term study of personality traits in patients with intractable obsessional illness treated by capsulotomy. *Acta Psychiatr Scand*, **99**, 40–50.

Nuttin, B., Cosyns, P., Demeulemeester, H., Gybels, J., & Meyerson, B. 1999. Electrical stimulation in anterior limbs of internal capsules in patients with obsessive-compulsive disorder. *Lancet*, **354**, 1526.

Oh, M. Y., Abosch, A., Kim, S. H., Lang, A. E., & Lozano, A. M. 2002. Long-term hardware-related complications of deep brain stimulation. *Neurosurgery*, **50**, 1268–74; discussion 74–6.

Okun, M. S., Bowers, D., Springer, U., Shapira, N. A., Malone, D., Rezai, A. R., Nuttin, B., Heilman, K. M. Morecraft, R. J., Rasmussen, S. A., Greenberg, B. D., Foote, K. D., & Goodman, W. K. 2004. What's in a "smile?" Intra-operative observations of contralateral smiles induced by deep brain stimulation. *Neurocase*, **10**, 271–9.

Paluzzi, A., Belli, A., Bain, P., Liu, X., & Aziz, T. M. 2006. Operative and hardware complications of deep brain stimulation for movement disorders. *Br J Neurosurg*, **20**, 290–5.

Sansur, C. A., Frysinger, R. C., Pouratian, N., et al. 2007. Incidence of symptomatic hemorrhage after stereotactic electrode placement. *J Neurosurg*, **107**, 998–1003.

Shapira, N. A., Okun, M. S., Wint, D., et al. 2006. Panic and fear induced by deep brain stimulation. *J Neurol Neurosurg Psychiatry*, **77**, 410–2.

Chapter 1

Transcranial Magnetic Stimulation (rTMS)

Eran Chemerinski, MD

Basic Concepts

Overview

Transcranial magnetic stimulation (TMS) is a noninvasive tool to modulate cortical excitability. The science behind it goes back to 1832, when Faraday demonstrated that changing magnetic fields can generate electrical currents. Using this principle of electromagnetism, Barker et al. (1985) used a single pulse magnetic device to stimulate the human cortex and spinal cord. This early single pulse-TMS technology continues to be used today for research and diagnostic purposes (i.e., nerve conduction studies). A decade later, modern repetitive TMS (rTMS) devices capable of generating rapid succession of magnetic pulses were developed. The recognition of the ability of rTMS to modulate (i.e., increase or decrease) the excitability of the brain cortex for extensive periods following stimulation sessions, led to the widespread use in various cognitive, psychiatric, and neurologic disorders. Despite the rising clinical adoption of the technique, most of the claims of efficacy of rTMS in disease states require further support from evidence-based data. Many rTMS outpatient clinics have been set up in the U.S. since the approval by the Food and Drug Administration (FDA) of the first rTMS device for the treatment of patients with medication-refractory depression in 2008. It is reasonable to anticipate continuous growth in the number of these clinics since, in contrast to other brain stimulation techniques that are either invasive such as deep brain stimulation (DBS), or require a seizure for their therapeutic effect such as electroconvulsive therapy (ECT), no anesthesia or recovery staff and space is involved in the provision of rTMS (Pridmore and Belmaker, 1999).

Theory of Mechanism of Action

rTMS devices are capable of generating a magnetic field from electric energy stored in a capacitor. This magnetic field penetrates the scalp and skull and

Brain Stimulation in Psychiatry: ECT, DBS, TMS, and Other Modalities, Charles H. Kellner. Published by Cambridge University Press. © Charles H. Kellner, 2012.

induces an electric field in the brain. The flow of ions created by this field alters the electric charges of cell membranes leading to neuronal depolarization or hyperpolarization. Initial insight into the mechanism of action of TMS comes from the observation that a single magnetic pulse from a coil applied to the scalp over the hand representation of the human primary motor cortex, depolarizes corticospinal tract neurons and triggers contralateral hand muscle movements (Pascual-Leone et al., 1996).

The physiological principles of rTMS are identical to single-pulse TMS. However, while single TMS pulses produce effects that are measured in milliseconds, repetitively applied pulses are hypothesized to result in lasting alterations of cortical function and behavior (Hallett, 2000). Currently available rTMS devices are capable of delivering pulses with frequencies of up to 20 cycles per second (i.e., Hertz or Hz). By convention, these frequencies have been characterized as slow (i.e., low frequency) and fast (i.e., high frequency). Slow rTMS stimulation refers to stimulation at frequencies of 5 Hz or less, while fast rTMS refers to the use of stimulation frequencies greater than 5 Hz. Evidence indicates that slow rTMS stimulation leads to transient reduction in local cortical activity (Chen et al., 1997). More selective stimulation of the inhibitory GABA neurons by low frequency rTMS could explain this phenomenon. In contrast, fast rTMS stimulation is associated with increased neuronal excitability (Pascual-Leone et al., 1994). Although not consistently observed, these distinctive effects of rTMS have clear therapeutic implications. In a double-blind, placebo-controlled, crossover study evaluating the antidepressant effect of daily rTMS over the left prefrontal cortex, Speer et al. (2000) reported that treatment with high-frequency rTMS (20 Hz) increased and low frequency rTMS (1 Hz) decreased regional cerebral blood flow (rCBF) in frontal and related subcortical circuits. Findings from electrophysiological and neuroimaging studies suggest that the effects of rTMS are not limited to the site of stimulation, but are likely to propagate to functionally linked areas, including subcortical brain regions (Maertens de Noordhout, 2006).

The use of daily prefrontal rTMS to treat depression stemmed from findings of frontal hypometabolism observed in some depressed individuals and from models of mood dysregulation caused by imbalances in the relationship between the prefrontal cortex and limbic regions. Thus it was postulated that mood improvement could be induced with rTMS from repeated sub-convulsive stimulations of the prefrontal cortex, which in turn would elicit increased activity in circuits involving regulatory pathways interacting with the limbic system (George, 2010). Moreover, following reports from functional imaging studies showing that in Major Depressive Disorder (MDD), the left prefrontal cortex is less active than the right, most authors assessing the efficacy of rTMS in this disorder have used high stimulation frequencies over the left dorsolateral prefrontal cortex (DLPFC).

At a molecular level, rTMS applied to the left DLPFC was found to induce the release of endogenous dopamine from the left caudate as a consequence of direct corticostriatal axon stimulation (Strafella et al., 2001) and of serotonin in hippocampal areas (Post and Keck, 2001). rTMS was reported to have similar effects as those of ECT, including the normalization of the hypothalamic-pituitary-adrenal (HPA) axis and a surge in the levels of brain-derived neuro-trophic factor (BDNF) and monoaminergic turnover (Yukimasa et al., 2006). Nevertheless, the physiological basis by which rTMS induces lasting effects on the brain and provides symptomatic relief of depression and other neuro-psychiatric illnesses has not been identified.

Patient Selection and Preparation

Indications

Depression

rTMS devices have been approved for the treatment of depression by regulatory agencies in Canada, Australia, New Zealand, Israel, Brazil, and the European Union. In the United States, the FDA granted the approval in 2008 of an rTMS device, the NeuroStar TMS Therapy® manufactured by Neuronetics, Inc., for the treatment of MDD in adult patients who have failed to achieve satisfactory improvement from one prior antidepressant medication at or above the min-imal effective dose and duration in the current episode. This decision was in large part based on results of an industry-sponsored, multisite, randomized clinical trial of 301 subjects with MDD who had previously failed to respond to at least one adequate antidepressant treatment trial and underwent either active (n = 155) or sham (n = 146) rTMS over the left DLPFC (O'Reardon et al., 2007b). Moreover, the parameters of stimulation approved by the FDA for the treatment of depression are those used in this study. The trial, which included 5 rTMS sessions a week for 4–6 weeks, used the following stimulation parame-ters: frequency of 10 Hz, 120% of motor threshold (MT), and 3,000 pulses/session. Results from this study indicated that active rTMS was significantly superior to sham rTMS for symptoms of depression scored by the Montgomery-Asberg Depression Rating Scale (MADRS) at week 4, as well as on the 17- and 24- item Hamilton Depression Rating Scale (HAM-D) at weeks 4 and 6. Response rates were significantly higher with active rTMS on all these scales at weeks 4 and 6. However, it is worth pointing out that while remission rates were approximately twofold higher with active rTMS compared to sham rTMS at week 6 (MADRS: 14.2% vs. 5.2%; HAM-D17: 15.5% vs. 7.1%; HAM-D24: 17.4% vs. 8.2%) these rates are far lower than those of other antidepressant treatments. Active rTMS was well tolerated with a low (4.5%) dropout rate for mild adverse events.

Among all neuropsychiatric disorders, the effectiveness of rTMS has been most widely studied in depression. Early studies reported relief of depressive symptoms with the use of high-frequency rTMS at 90% of motor threshold applied over the left DLPFC (Pascual-Leone and Catalá, 1996). Since then, most studies examining the effectiveness of rTMS on MDD have used high-frequency stimulation over this area. A meta-analytical review of these studies by Martin et al. (2003) suggests that the antidepressant effects of a 2-week course of rTMS over this cortical area are statistically superior to sham treatment. However, findings from these studies are difficult to compare due to the use of a great variety of stimulation parameters and study designs as well as heterogeneous depressed populations, small sample sizes, and dubious sham controls.

The duration of treatment in rTMS trials of MDD has progressively increased over time to up to 6 weeks, or even longer. The intensity of rTMS stimulation, number of pulses and daily stimulation trains are also higher in recent studies compared to earlier ones (Daskalakis et al., 2008). In a meta-analytical review, Gross et al. (2007) hypothesize that the better outcomes reported by more recent rTMS trials of MDD are explained by these higher doses.

Alternative stimulation sites and frequencies have been examined in rTMS trials of depression. In a study by Klein et al. (1999), 70 patients with MDD were randomly assigned to receive right prefrontal sham or active low frequency (1 Hz) rTMS stimulation during a 2-week period. At the end of the treatment period, 17 of 35 (49%) patients in the rTMS group, but only 8 of 32 (25%) in the sham-treated group experienced >50% mood improvement measured by the 17-item HAM-D and the MADRS. The authors concluded that this finding provides evidence for the short-term efficacy of slow rTMS in MDD patients. More recently, several non-industry multisite rTMS depression trials, including one sponsored by the National Institutes of Health (George et al., 2010), have been undertaken to evaluate not only previous reports of effectiveness of rTMS in the acute phase of depression, but to examine its effectiveness as a maintenance treatment for this disorder.

rTMS has also been used to treat depression associated with neurological conditions. For example, a study by Jorge et al. (2004) found that 10 sessions of active, high-frequency rTMS of the left DLPFC were associated with a significant reduction of depressive symptoms in patients with post-stroke depression who had not responded to antidepressants. This finding is important because depression has been shown to considerably impact recovery and mortality in post-stroke patients.

Posttraumatic Stress Disorder

rTMS stimulation of the right DLPFC at high frequencies, has been reported to reduce symptoms of posttraumatic stress disorder (PTSD). Reports from a double-blind, placebo-controlled investigation (Cohen et al., 2004) on 24 patients with PTSD randomly assigned to receive 10 daily sessions over 2 weeks of sham rTMS or either low frequency (1 Hz) or high-frequency (10 Hz) rTMS at 80% of the motor threshold over the right DLPFC, indicated that the core symptoms of this disorder (re-experiencing and avoidance) markedly improved in those subjects who received high-frequency rTMS. In a different double-blind, sham-controlled cross over study of low-frequency rTMS (1 Hz) over the right DLPFC, the hyperarousal symptoms of PTSD showed greater improvement with active stimulation compared to sham treatment (Osuch et al., 2009). However, further sham-controlled trials of rTMS for PTSD are needed. rTMS has not yet gained approval for the clinical treatment of PTSD.

Obsessive-Compulsive Disorder

An early study by Greenberg et al. (1997) suggested that rTMS over the right DLPFC might affect prefrontal mechanisms involved in obsessive-compulsive disorder (OCD). In this study, 12 patients with OCD were randomized to receive rTMS stimulation (80% MT, 20 Hz, 2 seconds per minute for 20 minutes) to the right DLPFC, left DLPFC and mid-occipital area on different days. Compulsive urges decreased significantly for 8 hours in patients who received rTMS over the right DLPFC. However, this reduction was shorter-lasting (30 minutes) and nonsignificant after left DLPFC rTMS stimulation. More recent double-blind placebo-controlled studies failed to show any therapeutic benefit of rTMS in OCD, either alone or combined with antidepressant medication (Sachdev et al., 2007; Prasko et al., 2006). A recent review of all studies of rTMS in the treatment of OCD from 1966 to 2010 (Jaafari et al., 2011) found that rTMS over the DLPFC is not significantly effective when compared to sham rTMS. The authors of this study suggest that because the available data are quite heterogeneous in terms of sample size, study design, stimulus parameters, and stimulation areas targeted, larger randomized, controlled trials should be conducted to better clarify the therapeutic role of rTMS in OCD.

Schizophrenia

Auditory hallucinations (AH) are hypothesized to be associated with hyperactivity of the left temporoparietal cortex (TPC). Thus, several research groups have used low frequency stimulation over this area to treat AH of schizophrenia. In a study by Hoffman et al. (2003), 24 patients with schizophrenia and schizoaffective disorder with medication resistant AH received low frequency (1 Hz) rTMS to the left TPC for 9 days. Half of these patients experienced a significant reduction in the frequency of AH that lasted for more than 3 months. However, a recent review of rTMS studies of schizophrenia (Poulet et al., 2010; Aleman et al., 2007) reported that this therapeutic action of rTMS is largely transient. Additionally, not all features of AH respond equally to rTMS. While some authors found significant rTMS treatment effects for *frequency* of AH (Hoffman et al., 2005; Lee et al., 2005), others found a significant treatment effect only for *loudness* of voices (Fitzgerald et al., 2005).

Negative symptoms of schizophrenia have been associated with prefrontal hypoactivity and only partially respond to medication. Prikryl et al. (2007)

applied 15 sessions of high-frequency (10 Hz) or sham rTMS over the left PFC of patients with schizophrenia and prominent negative symptoms. A significant decrease in these symptoms 29% reduction in the Positive and Negative Symptom Scale (PANSS) negative symptom subscale and 50% reduction in the Scale for the Assessment of Negative Symptoms (SANS), was found in the active rTMS group compared to the sham group. Conversely, Fitzgerald et al. (2008) and Barr et al. (2011) failed to show significant improvement in these symptoms with bilateral PFC rTMS.

Mania

The data on the effectiveness of rTMS in mania should be interpreted with caution because they derive mainly from open case series of patients on concomitant psychotropic medication during rTMS treatment. In an open label study by Saba et al. (2004), 8 medicated manic bipolar patients received five trains of 15-second, 10 Hz rTMS stimulation at 80% of the motor threshold over the right DLPFC. At the end of the trial, patients experienced a significant improvement of manic symptoms measured by the Mania Assessment Scale (MAS) and the Clinical Global Impression (CGI) scale. In another open label study by Michael and Erfurth (2004), 8 manic bipolar I inpatients received right DLPFC rTMS as add-on treatment to an only partially effective mood stabilizer and antipsychotic medication regimen. A sustained reduction in manic symptoms, as measured by the Bech-Rafaelsen Mania Scale (BRMAS), was observed in all patients during the 4 weeks of rTMS treatment. However, the authors acknowledged that a clear causal relationship between the rTMS treatment and reduction of manic symptoms could not be established, due to the open and add-on design features of the study. More recently, Praharaj et al. (2009) reported that, in 41 medicated bipolar mania patients who were randomized to receive daily sessions of active or sham rTMS over the right DLPFC for 10 days, rTMS was well tolerated and significantly effective in improving manic symptoms as measured by the Young Mania Rating Scale (YMRS). In this study, the active rTMS group (n = 21) was comparable to the sham group (n = 20) with respect to age of onset of first episode, number of manic and depressive episodes, duration of the current episode, and pharmacological profile. However, all patients receiving add-on active rTMS achieved remission, compared with 65% receiving sham stimulation.

Attention Deficit Hyperactivity Disorder

rTMS has also been explored for the treatment of ADHD, a developmental disorder hypothesized to result from right hemisphere fronto-striatum-cerebellum circuit abnormalities. However, reports of effectiveness of rTMS in this disorder are scarce and anecdotal. Niederhofer (2008) reported that the application of 1 Hz rTMS for 5 days in the supplementary motor area (SMA) of a subject with ADHD resulted in significant improvement that lasted for at least

4 weeks. More recently, Bloch et al. (2010) attempted to explore the effectiveness of rTMS in ADHD in a double-blind, randomized study of 13 patients with ADHD who received either a single session of sham or high-frequency rTMS over the right prefrontal cortex. In this study, a significant beneficial effect on attention, but no effect on mood and anxiety, was observed 10 minutes after treatment, only in patients in the active rTMS group.

Headache

Headache is one of the most common side effects of rTMS. However, an incidental reduction of preexisting headache pain was observed in patients with MDD during and after receiving rTMS (O'Reardon et al., 2007a). Thus, rTMS may be beneficial in those patients who suffer from comorbid headaches and mood disorders. In migraine, the effects of rTMS are controversial. Migraines with auras are associated with brain hyperexcitability involving the occipital cortex. Since low-frequency rTMS has been shown to decrease neural excitability, a recent placebo-controlled blinded study examined the effectiveness of 1 Hz rTMS stimulation on 5 consecutive days over the vertex in 27 patients with migraines (Teepker et al., 2010). The number of days with migraine attacks during 8 weeks was significantly reduced from 9.36 ± 2.82 days to 6.79 ± 4.28 days in patients who received active treatment (n = 14). In the placebo group (n = 13), the number of migraine attacks also decreased, but not significantly. These findings indicate that, while rTMS treatment does not provide adequate prophylaxis, it might be associated with positive effects on the frequency of migraine attacks. Paradoxically, although high-frequency rTMS is associated with brain hyperexcitability, reports from a small pilot study suggest that high-frequency rTMS over the left DLPFC may also ameliorate migraines (Brighina et al., 2004).

Epilepsy

Several studies have examined the effectiveness of rTMS as an alternative approach to reduce seizure frequency in patients with refractory epilepsy. In an open-label study of 12 patients with epilepsy, two weeks of rTMS at 0.5 Hz over the epileptic focus was found to decrease the number of seizures, without reduction in interictal epileptiform discharges (Santiago-Rodriguez et al., 2008). More recently, Sun et al. (2011) reported that low-frequency rTMS (3 sessions per day, 0.5 Hz, 90% of motor threshold, and 500 pulses each session) in 17 patients with refractory partial epilepsy led to a decrease in seizure frequency and EEG epileptic discharges in the post-treatment period, as well as to improvement in the "psychological condition" of these patients evaluated with the Symptom Checklist-90, a scale that includes indices of somatization, depression, and anxiety. Because stimulation frequencies above 1 Hz can increase the activity of the motor cortex, the safety of rTMS in this especially seizure-prone population warrants further evaluation.

Parkinson's Disease

Alterations of the neuronal activity of the SMA play a crucial role in the pathophysiology of the abnormal motor symptoms of Parkinson's disease (PD). rTMS can modulate cortical activation in the SMA, and thus may have a role in treating PD. High-frequency rTMS applied over the SMA has been shown to provide relief of bradykinesia in PD (Hamada et al., 2009). Low-frequency rTMS applied over the same area led to a reduction of dyskinesia induced by long-term levodopa therapy for PD (Koch, 2010). However, this reduction was only transient and repeated sessions of rTMS were not effective in inducing persisting clinical benefits. Moreover, in 10 patients with PD who had low-frequency (1 Hz) trains delivered over the motor cortex for 4 consecutive days, neither total motor scores nor subscores for axial symptoms, rigidity, bradykinesia, and tremor showed any significant difference (Filipovic et al., 2010).

Tic Disorders

The use of low-frequency rTMS over the SMA has also been proposed for the treatment of tic disorders. An open label study by Kwon et al. (2011) reported that tic symptoms significantly improved in 10 children with Tourette syndrome after 10 daily sessions of 1 Hz rTMS over the SMA. However, the effectiveness of rTMS in tic disorders has not been demonstrated in larger randomized studies. For example, in a single-blind, placebo-controlled, cross-over rTMS trial of 16 patients with Tourette syndrome who received, in random sequence, 1 Hz motor, premotor, and sham rTMS, no significant improvement in symptoms was found after any of the rTMS conditions, as assessed by the Motor and Vocal Tic Evaluation Survey (Münchau et al., 2002).

Tinnitus

Clinical, neurophysiologic and neuroimaging data suggest that chronic tinnitus is characterized by focal brain activation. In a functional imaging examination of a patient suffering from tinnitus, Langguth et al. (2003) found increased metabolic activity of the left primary auditory cortex. In this patient, tinnitus improved remarkably for several weeks after the use of low frequency (1 Hz) rTMS over this area for 4 weeks. More recently, Minami et al. (2011) applied a single session of low-frequency (1 Hz) rTMS over the left auditory cortex in 16 patients with chronic tinnitus. Seven of these patients experienced a significant (>20%) reduction of loudness and annoyance of tinnitus measured by visual analog scales that persisted for one week. In a randomized, prospective, placebo-controlled study by Anders et al. (2010), 52 right-handed patients were treated with sham or active 1 Hz frequency rTMS over the auditory cortex for a period of two weeks. A significant reduction of symptoms compared to baseline was seen at the end of the treatment period in both active and sham rTMS groups. However, symptom improvement persisted for another 14 weeks only in the active rTMS group. In contrast to previous studies, a 10-day trial of *high*-frequency rTMS over the left temporoparietal cortex was found to be more beneficial than either sham or low-frequency (1 Hz) rTMS at 1-year follow-up in 66 patients with chronic tinnitus (Khedr et al., 2009).

rTMS in Specific Populations

Adolescents

While the efficacy of rTMS in depressed adults is supported by a growing body of research, few studies have examined this treatment modality in depressed pediatric populations. In fact, the focus of most pediatric rTMS studies has been on the treatment of ADHD, tic disorders and medication-resistant epilepsy. The major concern regarding the use of rTMS in pediatric populations is the risk of seizure, because the seizure threshold of children and adolescents is lower than that of adults. However, in a review by Quintana (2005), no seizures were reported in 1,036 children and adolescents (i.e., ages 2 weeks to 18 years) who underwent single-pulse TMS, paired-pulse TMS, and low and high-frequency rTMS.

While MDD is a common in adolescents, response rates to antidepressant medications and cognitive behavioral therapy are less than those observed in adults. Studies examining the use of high-frequency rTMS in small populations of depressed adolescents (Loo et al., 2006) have found it to be safe and moderately effective, either alone or in combination with medication and psychotherapy. In these patients, the most frequently reported adverse effect was mild headache.

Pregnancy

Several case reports (Nahas et al., 1999; Zhang et al., 2010) suggest that rTMS is a promising alternative for the treatment of MDD during pregnancy. More recently, Kim et al. (2011) found that 7 of 10 pregnant women with MDD in their second or third trimester experienced a decrease of >50% in HAM-D scores after 20 sessions of 1 Hz rTMS at 100% of motor threshold to the right DLPFC. Importantly, there were no adverse pregnancy or fetal outcomes observed in these women.

Depression affects up to 15% of women in the postpartum period. However, many of these women avoid antidepressant medications due to concerns about exposure of their newborn through breastfeeding. While ECT is an established safe and effective treatment in these patients, rTMS has been proposed as a less invasive, non-psychopharmacological alternative. A recent study by Garcia et al. (2010) reported that among 9 antidepressant medication-free women with postpartum depression (PPD), all achieved remission of symptoms after 20 rTMS treatments (10 Hz, 120% motor threshold) over the left DLPFC. At 6-month follow-up, 7 of these patients remained in remission despite the absence of further psychiatric intervention.

The Pre-rTMS Evaluation

Prior antidepressant treatment history should be thoroughly reviewed in all rTMS candidates. The FDA approval of rTMS as a clinical tool for depression is restricted to patients who have failed to achieve significant mood improvement with adequate doses of one antidepressant drug. The Antidepressant Treatment History Form (ATHF) is a clinical tool developed to assist clinicians in assessing patients' antidepressant history. Many patients with depression are exposed to treatment trials that are ineffective due to inadequate medication doses or treatment duration.

Another important part of the pre-rTMS assessment is the safety screening. This includes a review of contraindications, warnings, and precautions that should be considered for each candidate. Current rTMS devices are equipped with treatment coils that produce magnetic fields strong enough to affect nearby objects. Within 30 cm of the face of the treatment coil, the peak magnetic field can be greater than 5 Gauss, the recommended static magnetic field exclusion level for many electronic devices. Thus, patients should be screened for the presence of any devices or objects that contain electronics or ferromagnetic material whose performance might be affected by the rTMS system and could present a safety issue.

Contraindications

rTMS is *contraindicated* for use in patients who have non-removable conductive, ferromagnetic, or other magnetic-sensitive metals implanted within 30 cm of the treatment coil. Failure to follow this restriction could result in serious injury or death. Examples of vulnerable devices/objects include cochlear implants, ferromagnetic ocular implants, implanted electrodes or brain stimulators, aneurysm clips, stents, bullet fragments, EEG electrodes, CSF shunts, carotid stents, and facial tattoos with metallic ink. Conversely, standard amalgam dental fillings are not affected by the magnetic field and do not contraindicate treatment.

Although the magnetic field strength diminishes quickly with increasing distance from the coil, the use of rTMS in patients who have an implanted device that is activated or controlled by physiologic signals, even if located outside the 30 cm distance, could result in serious injury or death. These devices include pacemakers, vagus nerve stimulators, as well as implantable and wearable cardioverter-defibrillators.

Informed Consent

An important medicolegal issue is obtaining informed consent from all candidates before the initiation of rTMS therapy. In such a consent document, all relevant information on the nature of the procedure as well as its potential risks should be disclosed in a way that is understandable to the patient.

Technique

Technical Requirements

The hardware of the Neurostar rTMS equipment is comprised of a capacitor for energy storage and an electromagnetic coil. This coil is a triggering component that allows the discharge of the stored energy in the form of a localized brief pulse of magnetic field to the surface of the head. During the discharge, the electrostatic charge stored in the capacitor flows in the form of electrical current to the stimulating coil, where it is rapidly converted into magnetic energy. The main effect of this magnetic impulse is to depolarize neurons by inducing electric fields within the brain. The magnetic impulse generated by conventional rTMS devices of 1.5–2.0 Tesla is able to penetrate the brain and activate neural tissue. However, this field can only reach the portion of the cerebral cortex that lies on the brain surface (i.e., not exceeding a depth of up to 3 cm beneath the scalp).

Stimulating coils consist of copper wires and electronic circuits housed in a plastic enclosure. Temperature sensors and cooling components are also included in their structure to prevent overheating of the coil, a cause of significant limitation on effective and safe operation. Different coil shapes are presently available. Circular coils are versatile, but fail to deliver stimulation that is sufficiently focal or that penetrates deeply in the brain. Thus, to be able to generate more focal and deep stimulation, other types of coils have been designed. However, these coils are not without their own disadvantages. For example, large double cone coils generate stimulation that can penetrate neural tissue relatively deeply, but possess poor focality. Conversely, higher stimulation focality is delivered under the junction of coils with a figure 8 design. However, the efficiency of these coils is reduced by the accumulation of charge in components that are non-tangential to the scalp (Rossini et al., 2010).

rTMS treatments are delivered while patients sit in a treatment chair designed for maximum comfort and lumbar support (see Figure 10.1). This chair has an electro-mechanical head support system attached to it that is intended to provide a reliable coil position measurement for motor threshold determination and treatment location.

A fundamental component of the Neurostar rTMS equipment is its system software. The software of this device includes a proprietary application that guides system operation through the treatment procedure with the use of a work-flow management chart.

Procedure

Motor Threshold Determination

Motor threshold (MT) is usually defined as the minimum amount of energy needed to produce contraction of the contralateral abductor pollicis brevis muscle of the thumb when the rTMS coil is held over the hand area of the contralateral motor cortex. MT is a measure of general cortical excitability and a crucial parameter for the determination of rTMS dose intensities. Instead of using a universal absolute value, current rTMS studies set dosage intensity as a percentage of each patient's MT. In most therapeutic or research studies this intensity is approximately 80–120% of the individual's MT. The MT intensity level is initially determined for each new patient undergoing rTMS and subsequently when there has been a change in his/her medical condition or prescription medication.

Before the determination of MT, each patient's individual MT location has to be identified. The MT location or optimal site of stimulation in the scalp that elicits a contraction of the contralateral thumb varies among patients due to anatomical differences. This site is determined by positioning the coil at 5 cm from the vertex in a coronal plane and moving it to several places in the vicinity. During this process, the intensity of discharge used is around 70% of the device output. Once a contraction is observed, the intensity is decreased manually or automatically until the MT, or the lowest intensity able to induce a contraction in the contralateral muscle 50% of the time, is achieved. The patient's MT location will be used later as a point of reference to establish an optimal area to position the coil for the treatment. For example, the left DLPFC is most frequently targeted by positioning the rTMS coil at a location on the scalp situated 5 cm anterior from the spot used to elicit the MT.

Treatment Course

Although alternative treatment schedules have been proposed, typical rTMS treatments for depression are comprised of 20–40 minute sessions, 5 days a week (i.e., weekdays) for 4–6 weeks.

The treatment parameters of the presently FDA-approved rTMS device for therapeutic use (NeuroStar TMS), are programmed for each treatment session following these National Institute of Neurological Disorders and Stroke (NINDS) guidelines. Although the device has the ability to be set to other stimulation parameters, the manufacturer recommends following these guidelines to decrease the risk of seizures. The parameters are as follows: intensity: 120% of the patient's observed MT; frequency: 10 Hz; pulse repetition cycle: 30-second cycle, with a stimulation treatment train duration of 4 seconds, and an interval of 26 seconds. The use of these parameters results in treatment session durations of 37.5 minutes and 3,000 magnetic pulses administered per session.

Safety issues

Treatment parameters for individual sessions should follow current safety guidelines based on findings from rTMS studies that were performed more than a decade ago at the National Institute of Neurological Disorders and Stroke. Alarming reports of rTMS-induced seizures experienced by participants of the NINDS and other early studies led to the need to determine safe ways to deliver rTMS. For this purpose, leading researchers in the fields of psychiatry and neurophysiology gathered in 1996 at an international consensus workshop on the safety of rTMS. They established the maximum safe durations of single trains of rTMS at various frequencies and intensities based on the NINDS experience (Wassermann, 1998). Present safety guidelines allow for all slow rTMS pulses to be applied in a continuous stimulation train of up to 20 minutes at a time. However, these guidelines recommend that the trains for fast rTMS, should be shorter and separated by periods without stimulation (i.e., inter-train intervals).

Following these guidelines, the risks of rTMS are very low, as reviewed in recent meta-analyses of the published literature (Machii et al., 2006; Loo et al., 2008; Janicak et al., 2008). However, the expanding uses of rTMS compel the periodic reexamination of current safety recommendations. Similarly, fundamental matters such as who is competent to actually deliver rTMS have not yet been determined. It is expected that rTMS practitioners be competent in the basics of brain physiology and rTMS mechanisms, protocols and safety issues. Moreover, universal training guidelines and accreditation requirements for rTMS providers, beyond those offered by the manufacturers, are needed to ensure that this therapeutic tool is correctly and safely used (Horvath et al., 2011).

Maintenance Treatment

During rTMS therapy for depression, symptom improvement should be evaluated at regular intervals to determine when acute treatment is complete. Although in many cases mood improvement occurs before completion of the prescribed course, patients are urged to complete the full acute treatment course to prevent relapse. However, as occurs with other treatments for depression, some patients begin to relapse quickly after the acute course of rTMS treatment. Thus, investigators have explored the use of maintenance rTMS. O'Reardon et al. (2005) applied 1 to 2 weekly sessions of rTMS to the left PFC of 10 adults with unipolar depression for periods ranging from 6 months to 6 years. Seven of the 10 subjects experienced either marked or moderate benefit. However, this benefit was sustained without the addition of concomitant antidepressant medication in only 3 cases. Thus, further research into the long-term efficacy of rTMS is warranted. Alternative maintenance treatment schedules have been proposed. For example, a Canadian group has used an intensive monthly regimen (i.e., 5 treatments sessions provided over one weekend a month) as an effective rTMS maintenance schedule (Fitzgerald and Daskalakis, 2011).

Monitoring

Besides monitoring patients' clinical status, qualified clinicians should also examine their cognitive, sensory, and motor functions on a periodic basis before, during, and after rTMS treatment. An example of motor monitoring is the simple visualization by rTMS operators of contractions of patients' facial muscles during the stimulus application, which might indicate spread of excitation that can precipitate a seizure.

Concurrent Medications

Most clinicians recommend that patients continue taking their antidepressant medication(s) during the course of rTMS. Antidepressants should also be continued while tapering rTMS treatment. This practice is supported by reports from a recent study (Cohen et al., 2009) indicating that less than one quarter of a large group of depressed patients (n = 204) successfully treated with rTMS remained symptom free at their 6-month follow-up.

While the safety of rTMS treatment in conjunction with antidepressant medication has not been evaluated in controlled clinical trials, observations from patients who continued taking these drugs during the course of rTMS suggest that this practice is safe. Despite this, the treating physician should review each patient's medication history and determine whether or not it is clinically appropriate to administer rTMS in conjunction with their medication. Moreover, if a medication is administered concurrently with rTMS therapy, it is recommended that a motor threshold determination be performed before treatment sessions following dose changes.

Common Adverse Effects

Headache and Neck Pain

Tension-type headaches of mild-to-moderate severity are the most common adverse effects of rTMS. In a recent meta-analysis of sham-controlled studies, Machii et al. (2006) found that headaches were experienced by approximately 28% of subjects receiving active rTMS treatment. While headaches are hypothesized to result from the direct stimulation of superficial facial nerves (e.g., trigeminal) and muscles, up to 16% of subjects who received rTMS sham treatment also experienced this symptom. Thus, the cause of rTMS-induced headaches is uncertain. Additionally, the relationship between this symptom and rTMS stimulus intensity and frequency is unclear. For example, Loo et al. (2008) found headache severity to be associated with higher intensities and frequencies. However, a previous study by Machii et al. (2006) reported greater incidence of headache with low-frequency rather than high-frequency prefrontal rTMS (34% vs. 25%, respectively). Other factors such as individual susceptibility, coil design, and location of stimulus also have been hypothesized to play a role in the severity of headaches.

In addition to headaches, a significant number of individuals treated with rTMS also experience neck pain, which may result from the forced immobilization of the head to optimize contact with the coil during the rTMS session. Nevertheless, because rTMS-induced headaches and neck pain promptly subside with or without the use of simple analgesics, discontinuation of treatment due to pain only occurs in a very small number of patients (Janicak et al., 2008). Several strategies to reduce rTMS-induced pain have been explored. For example, some authors recommend the use of a treatment algorithm that starts below target dose and increases gradually over the first week of treatment. Additionally, Borckardt et al. (2006) reported that a local injection of lidocaine significantly reduced pain intensity during rTMS treatment. In this study, 2 subjects identified the scalp area of maximum discomfort during stimulation with 6 trains of baseline rTMS. After 1.5 ml of 2% lidocaine was injected in a fanlike distribution in the subcutaneous tissues of that area, these subjects experienced a significant reduction of pain and unpleasantness measured by visual analog scales in subsequent rTMS applications. However, this reduction was not observed with the use of a topical anesthetic.

Hearing

The rapid mechanical deformation of the TMS stimulating coil resulting from the current discharged into it produces a characteristic brief noise that may exceed the recommended OSHA safety levels for the auditory system. Initial concerns of the potential of rTMS to cause hearing loss were raised after reports of permanent increases in auditory thresholds in animals exposed to high stimulation intensities (Counter et al., 1990). However, supplemental studies by the same group showed that the use of earplugs fully prevented hearing damage in those animals exposed to the rTMS noise for long periods. The use of ear protection is also supported by numerous reports of lack of rTMS-induced auditory damage in humans when ear protection was used (Levkovitz et al., 2007; Folmer et al., 2006; Janicak et al., 2008). Conversely, transient increases in auditory thresholds with the use of high-frequency rTMS have been found in subjects who did not use earplugs (Pascual-Leone et al., 1992). Thus, while the factor that determines the risk of hearing loss has been disputed (i.e., intensity of the peak sound pressure level vs. overall duration of exposure), it is universally recommended that subjects undergoing rTMS be provided with approved hearing protection such as ear plugs. The rTMS operator and other individuals present in the room should also wear ear protection because the noise produced by rTMS is not mitigated by distance from the coil. Additional recommendations (Rossi et al., 2009) for the prevention of rTMS-induced hearing loss include the prompt referral for auditory assessment of all individuals who complain of hearing loss, tinnitus, or aural fullness during rTMS treatment, as well as the assessment of the risk/benefit ratio in individuals with known hearing loss or concurrent treatment with ototoxic medications. As noted above, the presence of cochlear implants is a contraindication for rTMS.

Seizures

The risk of accidentally inducing a seizure with rTMS is very low. This risk is elevated when pulses are applied at high frequencies and with short intervals between trains of stimulation. A recent systematic review of all published rTMS studies (Rossi et al., 2009) identified only 4 subjects who suffered accidentally induced seizures while treated within the safe limit parameters of intensity, frequency, and duration suggested by the International Workshop on the Safety of rTMS (Wassermann, 1998). Of these subjects, 2 might have experienced non-epileptic events (i.e., pseudoseizure and convulsive syncope) instead of actual seizures. Additionally, 3 of these subjects were receiving concurrent pro-convulsant drugs. In contrast to reports of seizures occurring during or immediately after sessions, no conclusive evidence exists that rTMS causes tardive seizures. In fact, the decrease of cortical excitability induced by low-frequency rTMS has been examined as a way to suppress seizures in patients with epilepsy. In these patients, the risk of rTMS-induced seizures has also been found to be very low. In a recent review of studies from 1990 until 2007 in which rTMS was used for the treatment epilepsy, Bae et al. (2007) reported that a seizure occurred during treatment in only 4 cases. None of these events was life-threatening and the authors concluded that rTMS is nearly as safe in patients with epilepsy as in nonepileptic individuals. In any case, treatment with rTMS should always be performed according to safety guidelines (Wasssermann, 1998). In patients with additional risk (e.g., structural brain abnormalities), rigorous monitoring during treatment by a physician with expertise in the recognition and acute treatment of seizures is strongly recommended.

Psychiatric Adverse Effects

There have been numerous reports of psychiatric complications of rTMS. For example, Zwanzger et al. (2002) described a case of persecutory delusions triggered by high-frequency rTMS stimulation of the DLPFC in a medication-free depressed patient. While high-frequency rTMS stimuli of the right DLPFC has been shown to have therapeutic effects in mania (Erfurth et al., 2000), manic or hypomanic symptoms are the most frequently reported psychiatric complications of rTMS. Manic symptoms mostly occur in medication-free bipolar patients treated with high-frequency rTMS on the left DLPFC (Rachid and Bertschy, 2006). However, since rTMS-induced manic symptoms have also been shown to arise in patients treated with concurrent mood-stabilizing agents, all bipolar patients should be closely monitored for the emergence of these symptoms throughout the treatment course. DLPFC rTMS-induced mania has also been seen in subjects with unipolar depression (George et al., 1995) or without prior history of mood disorder (Nedjat and Folkerts, 1999). In all cases, manic or hypomanic symptoms promptly resolved with the cessation of rTMS or the addition of antimanic pharmacological agents.

Cognitive Effects

In contrast to ECT, no major cognitive effects have been reported among subjects who received rTMS. A study by O'Connor et al. (2003) compared the effects on mood and cognition in 14 patients with MDD who underwent treatment with unilateral ECT (3 times per week, for 2 to 4 weeks) vs. 14 patients with MDD treated with rTMS (stimulation over the left DLPFC, 90% of MT, 10 Hz, daily for 2 weeks). Results of this study indicated that ECT had a more positive effect on mood than rTMS. However, while patients treated with ECT experienced retrograde amnesia up to 2 weeks after treatment, there was no evidence of anterograde or retrograde memory deficits after rTMS. In a more recent study, the same research group (O'Connor et al., 2005) reported that performance on tasks of response speed and procedural memory improved in 19 patients with MDD examined following treatments with rTMS to the left DLPFC in daily sessions of 10 Hz stimuli at an intensity of 110% of the MT. No significant deterioration of cognitive performance was observed in a study that assessed the tolerability and safety of 10 Hz rTMS stimulation at 110% of MT over the left DLPFC in 32 medicated patients with schizophrenia (Mittrach et al., 2010).

The rTMS Service

Staffing and Administration

Physicians working in an rTMS service have responsibilities that go beyond the delivery of the treatment itself. These include designing an rTMS application protocol, overseeing the screening procedures to guarantee that candidates are assessed for risk factors and are provided with all necessary information about the treatment, and writing medical reports. Although rTMS treatment can only be prescribed by licensed physicians, its application can be carried out by properly trained medical technicians. A physician should be immediately available during the treatment, but his/her physical presence is not required in the rTMS treatment suite. Thus, it is essential that the medically responsible physician guarantee the proper training of rTMS operators working with him/her. To date, there is no official position about training requirements for these operators. While teaching courses are offered by public and private institutions, they are not presently mandatory. Training requirements should include practical training in the operation of the rTMS device, including stimulus settings and troubleshooting, basic knowledge of brain physiology as well as mechanisms of rTMS and physiological changes induced by it. Most importantly, physicians should make sure that medical assistants who will operate the rTMS device are properly trained in how to recognize and manage potential acute complications such as syncope and seizures.

Record Keeping

One of the most important aspects of medical record keeping is the protection of confidentiality of patient information. The Neurostar TMS device complies with Federal HIPAA regulations due to its capacity to record and store patients' data on a separate personal computer through the use of unique identifiers. Additional measures to protect these data include the use of wireless encryption programs and access to the system only by authorized providers through the use of name/password combinations. The patients' data electronically recorded is comprised of a *treatment session report* and a *patient therapy report*. The treatment session report is automatically generated at the end of each stimulation session and includes the identity of the operator and attending physician, number of pulses delivered, percentage of the patient's MT used, number of pulses per second (PPS), total stimulation time, length of intervals between pulses, and any modifications to the treatment. The patient therapy report can be generated at any time and includes items such as number of therapy sessions, MT level by date, and clinical rating type (e.g., HAM-D) and patient's score by date. Multiple other items such as medication types and doses and referring physician can be manually added to patients' electronic records.

The rTMS Suite

In medical centers, rTMS providers should comply with safety rules on rTMS determined by local authorities (IRB, Ethics Board, or Medical Board). However, in recent years there has been a significant growth in the number of rTMS treatment providers outside of medical settings. These settings are generally comprised of a treatment room with an adjacent waiting room. Treatment rooms should be large enough (at least 15 × 11 feet) to accommodate the rTMS device, (which includes a comfortable recliner where the patient sits during treatment), and allow the operator to work comfortably. Additionally, these rooms should be equipped with powerful air conditioning units to cool the coils and be soundproof and/or located away from areas where the loud tapping of the rTMS coil may be problematic. Most clinicians believe that due to the very low risk of severe adverse effects, rTMS can be carried out safely in these settings. However, because this risk is not completely absent, safety measures such as accessibility to appropriate life-support equipment and availability of the responsible physician should be ensured.

Conclusions

The clinical efficacy of rTMS remains controversial. rTMS treatment is usually well tolerated by patients, an important factor contributing to its rapid growth.

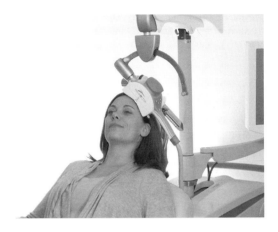

Figure 10.1. Patient set-up for TMS. Used with permission from Neuronetics, Inc.

Randomized, placebo-controlled, large-scale, multicenter trials are needed to determine if rTMS should be considered a standard therapeutic option for the treatment of depression and other neuropsychiatric disorders. Future research should help elucidate optimal cortical targets for stimulation as well as optimal stimulation parameters.

References

Aleman, A., Sommer, I., & Kahn, R. 2007. Efficacy of slow repetitive transcranial magnetic stimulation in the treatment of resistant auditory hallucinations in schizophrenia: a meta-analysis. *J Clin Psychiatry*, **68**, 416–21.

Anders, M., Dvorakova, J., Rathova, L., et al. 2010. Efficacy of repetitive transcranial magnetic stimulation for the treatment of refractory chronic tinnitus: a randomized, placebo controlled study. *Neuro Endocrinol Lett*, **31**, 238–49.

Bae, E., Schrader, L., Machii, K., et al. 2007. Safety and tolerability of repetitive transcranial magnetic stimulation in patients with epilepsy: a review of the literature. *Epilepsy Behav*, **10**, 521–8.

Barr, M., Farzan, F., Tran, L., Fitzgerald, P., & Daskalakis, Z. 2011. A randomized controlled trial of sequentially bilateral prefrontal cortex repetitive transcranial magnetic stimulation in the treatment of negative symptoms in schizophrenia. *Brain Stimul*, [Epub ahead of print].

Barker, A., Jalinous, R., & Freeston, I. 1985. Non-invasive magnetic stimulation of human motor cortex. *Lancet*, **1**, 1106–7.

Bloch, Y., Harel, E., Aviram, S., et al. 2010. Positive effects of repetitive transcranial magnetic stimulation on attention in ADHD Subjects: a randomized controlled pilot study. *World J Biol Psychiatry*, **11**, 755–8.

Borckardt, J., Smith, A., Hutcheson, K., et al. 2006. Reducing pain and unpleasantness during repetitive transcranial magnetic stimulation. *J ECT*, 22, 259–64.

Brighina, F., Piazza, A., Vitello, G., et al. 2004. rTMS of the prefrontal cortex in the treatment of chronic migraine: a pilot study. *J Neurol Sci*, 15, 67–71.

Chen, R., Classen, J., Gerloff, C., et al. 1997. Depression of motor cortex excitability by low-frequency transcranial magnetic stimulation. *Neurology*, 48, 1398–3.

Cohen, R., Boggio, P., & Fregni, F. 2009. Risk factors for relapse after remission with repetitive transcranial magnetic stimulation for the treatment of depression. *Depress Anxiety*, 26, 682–8.

Cohen, H., Kaplan, Z., Kotler, M., et al. 2004. Repetitive transcranial magnetic stimulation of the right dorsolateral prefrontal cortex in posttraumatic stress disorder: a double-blind, placebo-controlled study. *Am J Psychiatry*, 161, 515–24.

Counter, S., Borg, E., Lofqvist, L., & Brismar, T. 1990. Hearing loss from the acoustic artifact of the coil used in extracranial magnetic stimulation. *Neurology*, 40, 1159–2.

Daskalakis, Z., Levinson, A., & Fitzgerald, P. 2008. Repetitive transcranial magnetic stimulation for major depressive disorder: a review. *Can J Psychiatry*, 53, 555–66.

Erfurth, A., Michael, N., Mostert, C., & Arolt, V. 2000. Euphoric mania and rapid transcranial magnetic stimulation. *Am J Psychiatry*, 157, 835–6.

Filipovic, S., Rothwell, J., & Bhatia, K. 2010. Slow (1 Hz) repetitive transcranial magnetic stimulation (rTMS) induces a sustained change in cortical excitability in patients with Parkinson's disease. *Clin Neurophysiol*, 121, 1129–7.

Fitzgerald, P., Benitez, J., Daskalakis, J., et al. 2005. A double-blind sham-controlled trial of repetitive transcranial magnetic stimulation in the treatment of refractory auditory hallucinations. *J Clin Psychopharmacol*, 25, 358–62.

Fitzgerald, P., & Daskalakis, Z. 2011. The effects of repetitive transcranial magnetic stimulation in the treatment of depression. *Expert Rev Med Devices*, 8, 85–95.

Fitzgerald, P., Herring, S., Hoy, K., et al. 2008. A study of the effectiveness of bilateral transcranial magnetic stimulation in the treatment of the negative symptoms of schizophrenia. *Brain Stimul*, 1, 27–32.

Folmer, R., Carroll, J., Rahim, A., Shi, Y., & Hal Martin, W. 2006. Effects of repetitive transcranial magnetic stimulation (rTMS) on chronic tinnitus. *Acta Otolaryngol Suppl*, 556, 96–101.

Garcia, K., Flynn, P., Pierce, K., & Caudle, M. 2010. Repetitive transcranial magnetic stimulation treats postpartum depression. *Brain Stimul*, 3, 36–41.

George, M., Lisanby, S., Avery, D., et al. 2010. Daily left prefrontal transcranial magnetic stimulation therapy for major depressive disorder: a sham-controlled randomized trial. *Arch Gen Psychiatry*, 67, 507–16.

George, M., Wassermann, E., Williams, W., et al. 1995. Daily repetitive transcranial magnetic stimulation (rTMS) improves mood in depression. *Neuroreport*, 6, 1853–6.

George, M. 2010. Transcranial magnetic stimulation for the treatment of depression. *Expert Rev Neurother*, 10, 1761–2.

Greenberg, B., George, M., Martin, J., et al. 1997. Effect of prefrontal repetitive transcranial magnetic stimulation in obsessive-compulsive disorder: a preliminary study. *Am J Psychiatry*, **154**, 867–9.

Gross, M., Nakamura, L., Pascual-Leone, A., & Fregni, F. 2007. Has repetitive transcranial magnetic stimulation (rTMS) treatment for depression improved? A systematic review and meta-analysis comparing the recent vs. the earlier rTMS studies. *Acta Psychiatr Scand*, **116**, 165–73.

Hallett, M. 2000. Transcranial magnetic stimulation and the human brain. *Nature*, **406**, 147–50.

Hamada, M., Ugawa, Y., & Tsuji S. 2009. Effectiveness of rTMS on Parkinson's Disease Study Group, Japan. High-frequency rTMS over the supplementary motor area improves bradykinesia in Parkinson's disease: subanalysis of double-blind sham-controlled study. *J Neurol Sci*, **287**, 143–6.

Hoffman, R. E., Gueorguieva, R, Hawkins, K. A, Varanko, M., Boutros, N. N., Wu, Y. T., Carroll, K., & Krystal, J. H. 2005. Temporoparietal transcranial magnetic stimulation for auditory hallucinations: safety, efficacy and moderators in a fifty patient sample. *Biol Psychiatry*, **58**(2): 97–104.

Hoffman, R., Hawkins, K., Gueorguieva, R., et al. 2003. Transcranial magnetic stimulation of left temporoparietal cortex and medication-resistant auditory hallucinations. *Arch Gen Psychiatry*, **60**, 49–56.

Horvath, J., Perez, J., Forrow, L., Fregni, F., & Pascual-Leone, A. 2011. Transcranial magnetic stimulation: a historical evaluation and future prognosis of therapeutically relevant ethical concerns. *J Med Ethics*, **37**, 137–43.

Jaafari, N., Rachid, F., Rotge, J., et al. 2011. Safety and efficacy of repetitive transcranial magnetic stimulation in the treatment of obsessive-compulsive disorder: a review. *World J Biol Psychiatry*, [Epub ahead of print].

Janicak, P., O'Reardon, J., Sampson, S., et al. 2008. Transcranial magnetic stimulation in the treatment of major depressive disorder: a comprehensive summary of safety experience from acute exposure, extended exposure, and during reintroduction treatment. *J Clin Psychiatry*, **69**, 222–32.

Jorge, R., Robinson, R., Tateno, A., et al. 2004. Repetitive transcranial magnetic stimulation as treatment of poststroke depression: a preliminary study. *Biol Psychiatry*, **55**, 398–405.

Khedr, E.M, Rothwell, J.C., El-Atar, A. 2009. One-year follow up of patients with chronic tinnitus treated with left temporoparietal rTMS. *Eur J Neurol*, **16**, 404–8.

Kim, D. R., Sockol, L., Barber, J. P., Moseley, M., Lamprou, L., Rickels, K., O'Reardon, J. P., & Epperson, C. N. 2011. A survey of patient acdeptability of repetitive transcranial magnetic stimulation (TMS) during pregnancy. *J Affect Disord*. **129**, 385–90.

Klein, E., Kreinin, I., Chistyakov, A., et al. 1999. Therapeutic efficacy of right prefrontal slow repetitive transcranial magnetic stimulation in major depression: a double-blind controlled study. *Arch Gen Psychiatry*, **56**, 315–20.

Koch G. 2010. rTMS effects on levodopa induced dyskinesias in Parkinson's disease patients: searching for effective cortical targets. *Restor Neurol Neurosci*, **28**, 561–8.

Kwon, H., Lim, W., Lim, M., et al. 2011. 1-Hz low frequency repetitive transcranial magnetic stimulation in children with Tourette's syndrome. *Neurosci Lett*, **492**, 1–4.

Langguth, B., Eichhammer, P., Wiegand, R., et al. 2003. Neuronavigated rTMS in a patient with chronic tinnitus. Effects of 4 weeks treatment. *Neuroreport*, **14**, 977–80.

Lee, S. H., Kim, W., Chung, Y. C., Jung, K. H., Bahk, W. M., Jun, T. Y., Kim, K. S., George, M. S., & Chae, J. H. 2005. A double blind study showing that two weeks of daily repetitive TMS over the left or right temporoparietal cortex reduces symptoms in patients with schizophrenia who are having treatment-refractory auditory hallucinations. *Neurosci Lett*, **376**, 177–81.

Levkovitz, Y., Roth, Y., Harel, E., et al. 2007. A randomized controlled feasibility and safety study of deep transcranial magnetic stimulation. *Clin Neurophysiol*, **118**, 2730–44.

Loo, C., McFarquhar, T., & Walter, G. 2006. Transcranial magnetic stimulation in adolescent depression. *Australas Psychiatry*, **14**, 81–5.

Loo, C., McFarquhar T., & Mitchell, P. 2008. A review of the safety of repetitive transcranial magnetic stimulation as a clinical treatment for depression. *Int J Neuropsychopharmacol*, **11**, 131–47.

Machii, K., Cohen, D., Ramos-Estebanez, C., & Pascual-Leone, A. 2006. Safety of rTMS to non-motor cortical areas in healthy participants and patients. *Clin Neurophysiol*, **117**, 455–71.

Maertens de Noordhout, A. 2006. General principles for clinical use of repetitive transcranial magnetic stimulation (rTMS). *Neurophysiol Clin*, **36**, 97–103.

Martin, J., Barbanoj, M., Schlaepfer, T., et al. 2003. Repetitive transcranial magnetic stimulation for the treatment of depression. Systematic review and meta-analysis. *Br J Psychiatry*, **182**, 480–91.

Michael, N., & Erfurth, A. 2004. Treatment of bipolar mania with right prefrontal rapid transcranial magnetic stimulation. *J Affect Disord*, **78**, 253–7.

Minami, S., Shinden, S., Okamoto, Y., et al. 2011. Repetitive transcranial magnetic stimulation (rTMS) for treatment of chronic tinnitus. *Auris Nasus Larynx*, **38**, 301–6.

Mittrach, M., Thünker, J., Winterer, G., et al. 2010. The tolerability of rTMS treatment in schizophrenia with respect to cognitive function. *Pharmacopsychiatry*, **43**, 110–7.

Münchau, A., Bloem, B., Thilo, K., et al. 2002. Repetitive transcranial magnetic stimulation for Tourette syndrome. *Neurology*, **59**, 1789–91

Nahas, Z., Bohning, D., Molloy, M., et al. 1999. Safety and feasibility of repetitive transcranial magnetic stimulation in the treatment of anxious depression in pregnancy: a case report. *J Clin Psychiatry*, **60**, 50–2.

Nedjat, S., & Folkerts, H. 1999. Induction of a reversible state of hypomania by rapid-rate transcranial magnetic stimulation over the left prefrontal lobe. *J ECT*, **15**, 166–8.

Niederhofer, H. 2008. Effectiveness of the repetitive Transcranial Magnetic Stimulation (rTMS) of 1 Hz for Attention-Deficit Hyperactivity Disorder (ADHD). *Psychiatr Danub*, **20**, 91–2.

O'Connor, M., Brenninkmeyer, C., Morgan, A., et al. 2003. Relative effects of repetitive transcranial magnetic stimulation and electroconvulsive therapy on mood and memory: a neurocognitive risk-benefit analysis. *Cogn Behav Neurol*, **16**, 118–27.

O'Connor, M., Jerskey, B., Robertson, E., et al. 2005. The effects of repetitive transcranial magnetic stimulation (rTMS) on procedural memory and dysphoric mood in patients with major depressive disorder. *Cogn Behav Neurol*, 18, 223–7.

O'Reardon, J., Blumner, K., Peshek, A., Pradilla, R., & Pimiento, P. 2005. Long-term maintenance therapy for major depressive disorder with rTMS. *J Clin Psychiatry*, 66, 1524–8.

O'Reardon, J., Fontecha, J., Cristancho, M., & Newman, S. 2007a. Unexpected reduction in migraine and psychogenic headaches following rTMS treatment for major depression: a report of two cases. *CNS Spectr*, 12, 921–5.

O'Reardon, J., Solvason, H., Janicak, P., et al. 2007b. Efficacy and safety of transcranial magnetic stimulation in the acute treatment of major depression: a multisite randomized controlled trial. *Biol Psychiatry*, 62, 1208–16.

Osuch, E., Benson, B., Luckenbaugh, D., et al. 2009. Repetitive TMS combined with exposure therapy for PTSD: a preliminary study. *J Anxiety Disord*, 23, 54–9.

Pascual-Leone, A., & Catalá, M. 1996. Lateralized effect of rapid-rate transcranial magnetic stimulation of the prefrontal cortex on mood. *Neurology*, 46, 499–502.

Pascual-Leone, A., Rubio, B., Pallardó F., & Catalá M D. 1996. Rapid-rate transcranial magnetic stimulation of left dorsolateral prefrontal cortex in drug-resistant depression. *Lancet*, 348, 233–7.

Pascual-Leone, A., Valls-Solé, J., Wassermann, E., et al. 1992. Effects of focal transcranial magnetic stimulation on simple reaction time to acoustic, visual and somatosensory stimuli. *Brain*, 115, 1045–59.

Pascual-Leone, A., Valls-Solé, J., Wassermann, E., & Hallett, M. 1994. Responses to rapid-rate transcranial magnetic stimulation of the human motor cortex. *Brain*, 117, 847–58.

Post, A., & Keck, M. 2001. Transcranial magnetic stimulation as a therapeutic tool in psychiatry: what do we know about the neurobiological mechanisms? *J Psychiatr Res*, 35, 193–215.

Praharaj, S., Ram, D., & Aroroa, M. 2009. Efficacy of high frequency (rapid) suprathreshold repetitive transcranial magnetic stimulation of right prefrontal cortex in bipolar mania: a randomized sham controlled study. *J Affect Disord*, 117, 146–50.

Prasko, J., Paskova, B., Zalesky, R., et al. 2006. The effect of repetitive transcranial magnetic stimulation (rTMS) on symptoms in obsessive compulsive disorder. A randomized, double blind, sham controlled study. *Neuroendocrinol Lett*, 27, 327–32.

Pridmore, S., & Belmaker, R. 1999. Transcranial magnetic stimulation in the treatment of psychiatric disorders. *Psychiatry Clin Neurosci*, 53, 541–8.

Prikryl, R., Kasparek, T., Skotakova, S., et al. 2007. Treatment of negative symptoms of schizophrenia using repetitive transcranial magnetic stimulation in a double-blind, randomized controlled study. *Schizophr Res*, 95, 151–7.

Poulet, E., Haesebaert, F., Saoud, M., Suaud-Chagny, M., & Brunelin, J. 2010. Treatment of schizophrenic patients and rTMS. *Psychiatr Danub*, 22, S143–6.

Quintana, H. 2005. Transcranial magnetic stimulation in persons younger than the age of 18. *J ECT*, 21, 88–95.

Rachid, F., & Bertschy, G. 2006. Safety and efficacy of repetitive transcranial magnetic stimulation in the treatment of depression: a critical appraisal of the last 10 years. *Neurophysiol Clin*, **36**, 157–83.

Rossi, S., Hallett, M., Rossini, P., Pascual-Leone, A., & The Safety of TMS Consensus Group. 2009. Safety, ethical considerations, and application guidelines for the use of transcranial magnetic stimulation in clinical practice and research. *Clin Neurophysiol*, **120**, 2008–39.

Rossini, P., Rossini, L., & Ferreri, F. 2010. Brain-behavior relations: transcranial magnetic stimulation: a review. *IEEE Eng Med Biol Mag*, **29**, 84–95.

Saba, G., Rocamora, J., Kalalou, K., et al. 2004. Repetitive transcranial magnetic stimulation as an add-on therapy in the treatment of mania: a case series of eight patients. *Psychiatry Res*, **128**, 199–202.

Sachdev, P., Loo, C., Mitchell, P., McFarquhar, T., & Malhi, G. 2007. Repetitive transcranial magnetic stimulation for the treatment of obsessive compulsive disorder: a double-blind controlled investigation. *Psychol Med*, 37, 1645–9.

Santiago-Rodriguez, E., Cardenas-Morales, L., Harmony, T., Fernandez-Bouzas, A., Porras-Katz, E., & Hernandez, A. 2008. Repetitive transcranial magnetic stimulation decreases the number of seizures in patients with focal neocortical epilepsy. *Seizure*, 17, 677–83.

Speer, A., Kimbrell, T., Wassermann, E., et al. 2000. Opposite effects of high and low frequency rTMS on regional brain activity in depressed patients. *Biol Psychiatry*, **48**, 1133–41.

Strafella, A., Paus, T., Barrett, J., & Dagher, A. 2001. Repetitive transcranial magnetic stimulation of the human prefrontal cortex induces dopamine release in the caudate nucleus. *J Neurosci*, **21**, RC157.

Sun, W., Fu, W., Mao, W., Wang, D., & Wang, Y. 2011. Low-frequency repetitive transcranial magnetic stimulation for the treatment of refractory partial epilepsy. *Clin EEG Neurosci*, **42**, 40–4.

Teepker, M., Hötzel, J., Timmesfeld, N., et al. 2010. Low-frequency rTMS of the vertex in the prophylactic treatment of migraine. *Cephalalgia*, **30**, 137–44.

Wassermann, E. 1998. Risk and safety of repetitive transcranial magnetic stimulation: report and suggested guidelines from the International Workshop on the Safety of Repetitive Transcranial Magnetic Stimulation, June 5–7, 1996. *Electroencephalogr Clin Neurophysiol*, **108**, 1–16.

Yukimasa, T., Yoshimura, R., Tamagawa, A., et al. 2006. High-frequency repetitive transcranial magnetic stimulation improves refractory depression by influencing catecholamine and brain-derived neurotrophic factors. *Pharmacopsychiatry*, **39**, 52–9.

Zhang, X., Liu, K., Sun, J., & Zheng, Z. 2010. Safety and feasibility of repetitive transcranial magnetic stimulation (rTMS) as a treatment for major depression during pregnancy. *Arch Womens Ment Health*, **13**, 369–70.

Zwanzger, P., Ella, R., Keck, M., Rupprecht, R., & Padberg, F. 2002. Occurrence of delusions during repetitive transcranial magnetic stimulation (rTMS) in major depression. *Biol Psychiatry*, **51**, 602–3.

Magnetic Seizure Therapy (MST)

Introduction

Magnetic seizure therapy (MST) is an experimental brain stimulation technique that combines features of repetitive transcranial stimulation (rTMS) and ECT. It involves the induction of a cerebral seizure using a high-strength magnetic field, while the patient is under general anesthesia and muscle relaxation. Its development has been predicated on the assumption that a magnetically-induced seizure may have advantages in efficacy and tolerability, compared with an electrically induced seizure, because of better localization of site of initiation and focality of propagation.

Background and Overview

The quest to refine convulsive therapy has involved attempts to induce therapeutic seizures by various means: injected chemicals preceded electricity; even an inhaled gas (flurothyl or *Indoklon*) has been tried (Fink, 1979). Magnetic seizure induction is but the latest attempt to improve upon ECT technique.

As summarized by Rowny et al. (2009), "MST refers to the intentional induction of a seizure for therapeutic purposes using repetitive transcranial magnetic stimulation (rTMS). Thus, the devices that are used for MST are more powerful than the devices used in rTMS, in that they are capable of sustaining long stimulation trains at high frequencies for the purpose of controlled seizure induction inpatients under anesthesia. The aim of this experimental convulsive treatment is to achieve more focal seizure induction that would retain the proven efficacy of ECT in the treatment of depression, while reducing the cognitive side effects typically associated with ECT. The approach to realize this goal has been to take advantage of the focality of magnetic fields to more precisely target the brain circuitry believed to be involved in the pathogenesis of

Brain Stimulation in Psychiatry: ECT, DBS, TMS, and Other Modalities, Charles H. Kellner. Published by Cambridge University Press. © Charles H. Kellner, 2012.

depression, while sparing the neural circuitry implicated in the cognitive side effects."

A series of steps to develop MST from the conceptual level to its practical application in humans has been largely carried out by Lisanby and colleagues (Lisanby et al., 2001a, 2001b). These steps have included developing the technology necessary (adequately powerful devices that can be sufficiently cooled, appropriately shaped coils, etc.), safety testing in the primate model, and most recently, testing in human patients.

Neurophysiologic investigations demonstrate that seizure expression in MST is weaker, by various measures, than in ECT-induced seizures (Rowny et al., 2009).

MST in Depression

Lisanby et al. reported the first case of MST in a human in 2001 (Lisanby et al., 2001b). This was an open trial that demonstrated good antidepressant effect and tolerability in this patient. Kozel and colleagues reported the second case, again with good results in terms of tolerability and efficacy (Kosel et al., 2003). Ten depressed patients then participated in a study to demonstrate the safety of MST. The study design involved giving two MST sessions instead of ECT at the beginning of the course of treatment; subjects tolerated the MST sessions well. Subsequently, 20 patients were enrolled in a two-center trial designed to be the first demonstration of the antidepressant efficacy of a full course of MST, as well as to provide information on optimal MST stimulus characteristics (White et al., 2006). Patients received an average of 9 ECT sessions, and 53% had a greater than 50% decrease in depression rating scores.

Cognitive tolerability was, again, very good. Most recently, Kayser et al. (2011) randomized a total of 20 treatment-resistant depressed patients to receive either a course of right unilateral ECT or MST. Both groups showed significant and comparable decreases in depression ratings, good cognitive tolerability, and fairly comparable electroencephalographic seizure expression. The authors concluded that MST may be an alternative to ECT and called for larger-scale trials to confirm efficacy and safety.

Future Directions

MST is in the early experimental stages of clinical use. Questions remain about optimal dosimetry, site of stimulation and seizure induction, mechanism of action, and patient selection (Rowny et al., 2009). Despite these unknowns, MST shows promise: if it can combine the efficacy of ECT with a very benign cognitive effect profile, and it proves to be clinically feasible to administer, it may have role in clinical brain stimulation in the future.

References

Fink, M. 1979. *Convulsive Therapy: Theory and Practice*. New York: Raven Press.

Kayser, S., Bewernick, B. H., Grubert, C., et al. 2011. Antidepressant effects, of magnetic seizure therapy and electroconvulsive therapy, in treatment-resistant depression. *J Psychiatr Res*, **45**, 569–76.

Kosel, M., Frick, C., Lisanby, H. S., Fisch, H. U., & Schlaepfer, T. E. 2003. Magnetic seizure therapy improves mood in refractory major depression. *Neuropsychopharmacology*, **28**, 2045–8.

Lisanby, S. H., Luber, B., Finck, A. D., Schroeder, C., & Sackeim, H. A. 2001a. Deliberate seizure induction with repetitive transcranial magnetic stimulation in nonhuman primates. *Arch Gen Psychiatry*, **58**, 199–200.

Lisanby, S. H., Schlaepfer, T. E., Fisch, H. U., & Sackeim, H. A. 2001b. Magnetic seizure therapy of major depression. *Arch Gen Psychiatry*, **58**, 303–5.

Rowny, S. B., Benzl, K., & Lisanby, S. H. 2009. Translational development strategy for magnetic seizure therapy. *Exp Neurol*, **219**, 27–35.

White, P. F., Amos, Q., Zhang, Y., et al. 2006. Anesthetic considerations for magnetic seizure therapy: a novel therapy for severe depression. *Anesth Analg*, **103**, 76–80, table of contents.

Chapter 12

Vagus Nerve Stimulation (VNS)

Introduction

Vagus nerve stimulation (VNS), originally introduced as treatment for intractable epilepsy, has been used in psychiatric patients as adjunctive therapy for treatment-resistant depression. Its use in depression followed the serendipitous observation that mood improved in some epilepsy patients treated with VNS. Enthusiasm for this indication for VNS has waned, as its limited efficacy has become clearer. It may have an ongoing role in maintenance treatment for depression, but it is likely that VNS will be appropriate only for a very limited number of patients.

VNS consists of a pacemaker-like pulse generator device implanted in the upper chest wall and a wire wrapped around the left vagus nerve in the neck, tunneled subcutaneously to connect to the pulse generator. Thus, it requires an invasive surgical procure, typically performed by a vascular surgeon or neurosurgeon, to implant the device.

Background and Neurobiology

The vagus nerve, cranial nerve X, the longest cranial nerve, contains both afferent and efferent fibers. Cell bodies of the afferent fibers are located in the nodose ganglion and project to the nucleus of the tractus solitarius (NTS). Projections from the NTS involve the locus coeruleus and indirectly, multiple limbic brain regions. It is hypothesized that VNS works by stimulation of afferent vagus nerve fibers in the neck that affect brain regions critical in the regulation of mood. Stimulation of the vagus nerve is also thought to result in changes in neurotransmitters, including increases in GABA, norepinephrine, and serotonin, and a decrease in glutamate. The anticonvulsant effect of VNS, possibly related to its enhancement of GABA neurotransmission, may be related to its antidepressant effect, consistent with the use of anticonvulsant medication for the treatment of mood disorders (Swartz, 2009).

Brain Stimulation in Psychiatry: ECT, DBS, TMS, and Other Modalities, Charles H. Kellner. Published by Cambridge University Press. © Charles H. Kellner, 2012.

Studies in Depression

An open label multicenter pilot study of 30 patients with treatment resistant depression provided the initial evidence for efficacy in depression (Rush et al., 2000). In that study, 40% of patients showed reductions of at least 50% in their HAM-D scores, and 17% remitted. Interestingly, responders continued to improve over the 12 weeks of the study; this ongoing, sometimes delayed, response has been seen in later studies and is the basis for the optimism that VNS may be a viable maintenance treatment (Marangell et al., 2002; Nahas et al., 2005). The so-called "pivotal" trial that followed was a 10-week, randomized controlled, blinded design comparing active VNS with sham treatment, in which 210 outpatients with nonpsychotic major depressive disorder and 25 with bipolar depression participated. At 10 weeks, the response rate in the active group (n = 112) was 15.2%, vs. 10% in the sham group (n = 110). The authors concluded, "This study did not yield definitive evidence of short-term efficacy for adjunctive VNS in treatment-resistant depression." Despite the lack of compelling efficacy data, the U.S. Food and Drug Administration approved the Cyberonics VNS Therapy System as an adjunctive treatment for the indication of treatment-resistant depression in 2005.

Patient Selection

As noted by McClintock et al. in *Electroconvulsive and Neuromodulation Therapies* (Swartz, 2009), "Highly selective clinical decision making is appropriate for VNS prescription." Clearly, this modality should be reserved for severely ill patients with chronic treatment-resistant depression. Intolerance to antidepressant medication may be another factor in favor of consideration of VNS.

Interestingly, an implanted VNS device does not contradict the use of ECT. No complications were reported in the 14 patients in the "pivotal" trial who had ECT with VNS devices implanted (Burke and Husain, 2006). The VNS device was not affected by ECT. Because VNS is anticonvulsant, the device should be turned off before ECT.

VNS Device Stimulation Parameters

The VNS device is programmed by means of a wand held over the pulse generator. This is done in an outpatient setting. Parameters that can be set include: current, frequency, pulse width, and signal on and off time. The goal is to find settings that optimize efficacy and tolerability; to a certain extent, this is an empirical process based on trial and error.

Safety and Adverse Effects

Despite the fact that VNS device implantation requires a significant surgical procedure, it is quite safe. Adverse events may be divided into those related to the surgery and those related to the stimulation itself.

The stimulation may cause discomfort, cough or voice alteration (because of its effect on the recurrent laryngeal nerve). Such adverse effects may diminish over time and occur only when the stimulus is on (typically the stimulus would be on for 30 seconds and then off for 5 minutes) (Swartz, 2009). Stimulus parameters may be adjusted to diminish such annoying adverse effects.

There is limited information about explanation/revision of the VNS device (both leads and pulse generator) in patients who fail to benefit from the treatment or in whom some adverse event requires removal/revision of the device (Tran et al., 2011).

Conclusions

VNS is a novel, invasive procedure that has been successfully used as a treatment for refractory epilepsy and more recently for refractory depression. Although no life-threatening events occurred in the major clinical trials, only modest antidepressant benefit has been demonstrated. Because the risk-benefit ratio is unclear for many patients, we believe that the role of VNS for the treatment of depression and other psychiatric illness may be very limited in the future.

References

Burke, M. J., & Husain, M. M. 2006. Concomitant use of vagus nerve stimulation and electroconvulsive therapy for treatment-resistant depression. *J ECT*, **22**, 218–22.

Marangell, L. B., Rush, A. J., George, M. S., et al. 2002. Vagus nerve stimulation (VNS) for major depressive episodes: one year outcomes. *Biol Psychiatry*, **51**, 280–7.

Nahas, Z., Marangell, L. B., Husain, M. M., et al. 2005. Two-year outcome of vagus nerve stimulation (VNS) for treatment of major depressive episodes. *J Clin Psychiatry*, **66**, 1097–104.

Rush, A. J., George, M. S., Sackeim, H. A., et al. 2000. Vagus nerve stimulation (VNS) for treatment-resistant depressions: a multicenter study. *Biol Psychiatry*, **47**, 276–86.

Swartz, C. 2009. *Electroconvulsive and Neuromodulation Therapies*. New York: Cambridge University Press.

Tran, Y., Shah, A. K., & Mittal, S. 2011. Lead breakage and vocal cord paralysis following blunt neck trauma in a patient with vagal nerve stimulator. *J Neurol Sci*, **304**, 132–5.

Chapter 13

Transcranial Direct Current Stimulation (tDCS)

Transcranial Direct Current Stimulation

Transcranial direct current stimulation (tDCS) is a noninvasive brain stimulation technique that consists of applying a weak continuous electrical current via scalp electrodes. It was rediscovered about 10 years ago and has been the subject of much interest for the treatment of a wide variety of illnesses in recent years (Stagg and Nitsche, 2011). It remains experimental and of unclear clinical utility in psychiatric illness at this time.

Overview and Theoretical Background

The direct application of electrical currents to the scalp has a very long and checkered history, starting with the use of electric eels in ancient times, and developing in the 18th and 19th centuries with the invention of batteries. tDCS was tested in humans in the 1960s; in recent years clinical trials have begun to be published (Williams and Fregni in Swartz, 2009). The theory behind tDCS is that neuronal activity in cortical brain regions underlying the scalp electrodes may be modulated by applied electric currents. Functional brain imaging techniques now allow investigation of changes induced by the electrical current in brain (Zheng et al., 2011). An anode and a cathode placed on two locations on the scalp are required; the stimulating current may be up to 10 mA, but is typically in the range of 0.5–2 mA, applied over a time ranging from seconds to minutes. Electrodes may be made of sponge or cotton, often soaked in a saline solution.

Advantages of tDCS include portability of equipment, ease of use, and lack of serious adverse effects. The literature now comprises over 50 studies with several hundred subjects total, documenting its safety Williams and Fregni in (Swartz, 2009).

Clinical Uses

tDCS has been applied in stroke patients in an effort to stimulate lesioned cortex (Hummel and Cohen, 2005), in neuropsychological studies to enhance

Brain Stimulation in Psychiatry: ECT, DBS, TMS, and Other Modalities, Charles H. Kellner. Published by Cambridge University Press. © Charles H. Kellner, 2012.

cognition (Tanaka and Watanabe, 2009), in fibromyalgia (Fregni et al., 2006c), epilepsy (Fregni et al., 2006d), addictions (Boggio et al., 2008), pain syndromes (Fregni et al., 2006a), and Parkinson's disease (Fregni et al., 2006b).

Recent studies of tDCS in depression are of particular interest. Dell'osso and colleagues (Dell'osso et al., 2011) published the results of a trial in which 23 patients with pharmacotherapy-resistant depression received open label adjunctive tDCS for 5 days: 30% responded and 17% remitted. Martin et al. (2011) recently reported the results of a clinical trial in which 11 depressed patients who had failed tDCS with bifrontal electrodes were given 4 weeks of tDCS with fronto-extracephalic electrodes. Blinded ratings showed significant improvement in depressive symptoms, with excellent tolerability.

These preliminary study results indicate that there may a signal of anti-depressant efficacy for tDCS. Clearly larger, sham-controlled studies are needed. Stimulus location and stimulus parameters need to be further investigated, with the aim of increasing antidepressant efficacy.

It remains to be determined if tDCS will develop into a useful tool in the treatment toolbox of clinical psychiatry.

References

Boggio, P. S., Sultani, N., Fecteau, S., et al. 2008. Prefrontal cortex modulation using transcranial DC stimulation reduces alcohol craving: a double-blind, sham-controlled study. *Drug Alcohol Depend*, **92**, 55–60.

Dell'osso, B., Zanoni, S., Ferrucci, R., et al. 2011. Transcranial direct current stimulation for the outpatient treatment of poor-responder depressed patients. *Eur Psychiatry*, [Epub ahead of print].

Fregni, F., Boggio, P. S., Lima, M. C., et al. 2006a. A sham-controlled, phase II trial of transcranial direct current stimulation for the treatment of central pain in traumatic spinal cord injury. *Pain*, **122**, 197–209.

Fregni, F., Boggio, P. S., Santos, M. C., et al. 2006b. Noninvasive cortical stimulation with transcranial direct current stimulation in Parkinson's disease. *Mov Disord*, **21**, 1693–702.

Fregni, F., Gimenes, R., Valle, A. C., et al. 2006c. A randomized, sham-controlled, proof of principle study of transcranial direct current stimulation for the treatment of pain in fibromyalgia. *Arthritis Rheum*, **54**, 3988–98.

Fregni, F., Thome-Souza, S., Nitsche, M. A., et al. 2006d. A controlled clinical trial of cathodal DC polarization in patients with refractory epilepsy. *Epilepsia*, **47**, 335–42.

Hummel, F., & Cohen, L. G. 2005. Improvement of motor function with noninvasive cortical stimulation in a patient with chronic stroke. *Neurorehabil Neural Repair*, **19**, 14–9.

Martin, D. M., Alonzo, A., Mitchell, P. B., Sachdev, P., Galvez, V., & Loo, C. K. 2011. Fronto-extracephalic transcranial direct current stimulation as a treatment for major depression: an open-label pilot study. *J Affect Disord*, **134**, 459–63.

Stagg, C. J., & Nitsche, M. A. 2011. Physiological basis of transcranial direct current stimulation. *Neuroscientist*, **17**, 37–53.

Swartz, C. 2009. *Electroconvulsive and Neuromodulation Therapies*. New York: Cambridge University Press.

Tanaka, S., & Watanabe, K. 2009. (Transcranial direct current stimulation – a new tool for human cognitive neuroscience]. *Brain Nerve*, **61**, 53–64.

Zheng, X., Alsop, D. C., & Schlaug, G. 2011. Effects of transcranial direct current stimulation (tDCS) on human regional cerebral blood flow. *Neuroimage*, **58**, 26–33.

Epidural Cortical Stimulation (EpCS)

Introduction

Epidural cortical stimulation (EpCS) is a novel brain stimulation technique in which electrodes are attached to the dura to stimulate the underlying cortex. It is an invasive procedure, requiring a bone flap to be opened in the skull, but is less invasive than deep brain stimulation (DBS) because brain tissue does not have to be penetrated by the stimulating electrodes. To a large extent, it is modeled after repetitive transcranial magnetic stimulation (rTMS), in that it involves cortical stimulation of targeted brain areas hypothesized to be involved in, or connected to, brain areas involved in mood regulation. Advantages include the ability to provide continuous stimulation and eliminate the need for repeated visits to a clinical site for treatment, a major disadvantage of rTMS.

Technique

A craniotomy is performed under general anesthesia over the predetermined area of cortex, guided by a stereotactic device. The stimulating electrode is anchored epidurally (lying on the dura), by suturing it to the dura. The craniotomy bone flap is then secured in place and the electrode lead is tunneled underneath the scalp and skin of the neck and connected to a neuro-stimulator/battery implanted in the subclavicular area of the chest wall.

Clinical Trials in Depression

To date, there have been two clinical trials in depression. Additionally, EpCS has been used experimentally in movement disorders, post-stroke motor recovery, neuropathic pain, and tinnitus (Priori and Lefaucheur, 2007; Brown et al., 2006; Velasco et al., 2008; Friedland et al., 2007).

Nahas et al. enrolled 5 highly treatment-resistant depressed patients in a pilot trial to test the safety and potential therapeutic benefit of prefrontal epidural stimulation (Nahas et al., 2010). Cortical stimulation leads were placed

Brain Stimulation in Psychiatry: ECT, DBS, TMS, and Other Modalities, Charles H. Kellner. Published by Cambridge University Press. © Charles H. Kellner, 2012.

bilaterally over the anterior frontal poles and midlateral prefrontal cortex. Stimulation was intermittent, analogous to that given with rTMS. Results at 7 months were encouraging, with patients having approximately a 50% reduction in depression rating scores and 3 patients reaching remission. One patient required lead explantation of left hemisphere leads because of scalp infection.

Kopell et al. enrolled 12 patients in a single-blind, sham-controlled multi-center study of the safety and feasibility of chronic (104-week follow-up) epidural stimulation (Kopell et al., 2011). An electrode was implanted over the mid-portion of the left middle frontal gyrus, corresponding to Brodmann area 9/46. They, too, demonstrated substantial clinical improvement, with 5 patients showing greater than 50% improvement, and 4 achieving remission. Note that stimulation was continuous, as opposed to intermittent in the Nahas study. PET imaging, carried out at baseline and again after response or study week 28, showed that higher right dorsolateral prefrontal cortex (DLPFC) metabolic activity at baseline was a predictor of response and that EpCS led to higher metabolic activity in the DLPFC. One patient developed a bone flap infection and one patient suicided, underscoring the severe nature of the depressive illness being treated.

Conclusions

EpCS is a novel, invasive brain stimulation technique that is beginning to be used experimentally in psychiatric illness. It is less invasive than DBS and has the advantage over rTMS that is self-contained and does not require the daily clinic visits of current rTMS protocols. Much additional research, with well-designed, larger-scale clinical trials will be needed to determine whether EpCS will become a practically usable, clinical therapy for serious psychiatric illnesses. Neuroimaging studies may be helpful in guiding patient selection and elucidating the mechanism(s) of action of EpCS.

References

Brown, J. A., Lutsep, H. L., Weinand, M., & Cramer, S. C. 2006. Motor cortex stimulation for the enhancement of recovery from stroke: a prospective, multicenter safety study. *Neurosurgery*, **58**, 464–73.

Friedland, D. R., Gaggl, W., Runge-Samuelson, C., Ulmer, J. L., &Kopell, B. H. 2007. Feasibility of auditory cortical stimulation for the treatment of tinnitus. *Otol Neurotol*, **28**(8), 1005–12.

Kopell, B. H., Halverson, J., Butson, C. R., et al., 2011. Epidural cortical stimulation (EpCS) of the left dorsolateral prefrontal cortex for refractory major depressive disorder. *Neurosurgery*, **69**, 1015–29.

Nahas, Z., Anderson, B. S., Borckardt, J., et al., 2010. Bilateral epidural prefrontal cortical stimulation for treatment-resistant depression. *Biol Psychiatry*, **67**(2), 101–9.

Priori, A., & Lefaucheur, J. P. 2007. Chronic epidural motor cortical stimulation for movement disorders. *Lancet Neurol*, **6**(3), 279–86.

Velasco, F., Arguelles, C., Carrillo-Ruiz, J. D., et al., 2008. Efficacy of motor cortex stimulation in the treatment of neuropathic pain: a randomized double-blind trial. *J Neurosurg*, **108**(4), 698–706.

Index